MEDICINE MY VOCATION
FISHING MY RECREATION
Memoirs of a Physician and Flyfisherman

Other World Scientific Titles Edited by Gilbert Thompson

Nobel Prizes that Changed Medicine
ISBN: 978-1-84816-825-1
ISBN: 978-1-84816-826-8 (pbk)

Pioneers of Medicine Without a Nobel Prize
ISBN: 978-1-78326-383-7
ISBN: 978-1-78326-384-4 (pbk)

MEDICINE MY VOCATION FISHING MY RECREATION

Memoirs of a Physician and Flyfisherman

Gilbert Thompson
Imperial College London, UK

World Scientific

NEW JERSEY • LONDON • SINGAPORE • BEIJING • SHANGHAI • HONG KONG • TAIPEI • CHENNAI • TOKYO

Published by

World Scientific Publishing Europe Ltd.

57 Shelton Street, Covent Garden, London WC2H 9HE

Head office: 5 Toh Tuck Link, Singapore 596224

USA office: 27 Warren Street, Suite 401-402, Hackensack, NJ 07601

Library of Congress Cataloging-in-Publication Data
Names: Thompson, G. R. (Gilbert R.), author.
Title: Medicine my vocation, fishing my recreation : memoirs of a physician and flyfisherman / Gilbert Thompson, Imperial College London, UK.
Description: New Jersey : World Scientific, [2020] | Includes bibliographical references and index.
Identifiers: LCCN 2020001816 | ISBN 9781786348111 (hardcover) | ISBN 9781786348128 (ebook) | ISBN 9781786348135 (ebook other)
Subjects: LCSH: Physicians--Great Britain--Biography. | Fly fishing.
Classification: LCC R489.T749 A3 2020 | DDC 610.92 [B]--dc23
LC record available at https://lccn.loc.gov/2020001816

British Library Cataloguing-in-Publication Data
A catalogue record for this book is available from the British Library.

For any available supplementary material, please visit
https://www.worldscientific.com/worldscibooks/10.1142/Q0240#t=suppl

Desk Editors: Balasubramanian Shanmugam/Shi Ying Koe

Typeset by Stallion Press
Email: enquiries@stallionpress.com

Foreword by Sir Keith Peters FRS

The creation of an effective treatment for a life-threatening chronic disease is a rare event, usually achieved by the pharmaceutical or biotechnology industries at the cost of hundreds of millions of pounds. In this elegantly written autobiography, Gilbert Thompson describes how he revolutionised the treatment of familial hypercholesterolaemia, which leads to early death from cardiovascular disease — especially the heart attacks and strokes that result from the accumulation of cholesterol-rich deposits of atheroma in major arteries. In the mid-1970s at the Hammersmith Hospital in London, Thompson utilised the technique of plasma-exchange where the patient's high cholesterol plasma was substituted with a zero cholesterol plasma substitute, using the then recently developed blood-cell separator. This exchange treatment, repeated weekly or fortnightly for years, resulted in the regression of atheroma and established that cholesterol-induced vascular disease could be reversed if the cholesterol content of blood was sufficiently reduced. This "proof in principle" of the benefit of cholesterol lowering was applauded by experts in the lipid field, and stimulated interest in the potential of cholesterol-lowering drugs; and this in turn was given vital impetus by the work of the Japanese pharmacologist Akira Endo, whose discovery of the first of a group of drugs now known as statins, and their subsequent development by Merck Research Laboratories, Thompson describes authoritatively. The statin drugs are now recognised as being one of the major advances in medicine of the latter part of the 20th century, contributing importantly to the substantial reduction in arterial diseases that has been observed in recent decades.

The work of Thompson and his colleagues was initially met with widespread scepticism in the UK, especially by the cardiological establishment, with not insignificant help from the butter industry, who refused to believe that lowering blood cholesterol by dietary or other means was a useful approach to the prevention and treatment of cardiovascular disease. Particularly painful for Thompson was the opposition of the pioneering physician scientist Sir John McMichael FRS who had created at the Hammersmith what was probably the leading academic department of medicine in Europe and given Thompson a major career opportunity by appointing him to a junior post in his department. Thompson's description of the opposition by leading academic figures in the UK and the several decades of epidemiological studies and clinical trials that were needed to convince the sceptics makes compelling reading, and has sad topicality today as we struggle with anti-science lobbies such as those opposed to vaccination and the prevention of global warming.

Thompson's character jumps from the pages of the book and gives insight into his success as a resolute defender of a controversial field. Earlier, in order to devote his career to clinical lipidology he gave up a secure tenured appointment in a leading academic unit at the Hammersmith. Prior to that as a young Army doctor in Ghana he built a homemade apparatus to research genetic variants in blood haemoglobin, and in late middle age took up marathon running. But the book is also about his passion for flyfishing, of which I know little, but where I glimpse similarities between the need to be patient in sometimes uncomfortable circumstances and make intelligent and informed decisions about where to cast the fly, with no guarantee of reward, and what medical researchers experience as they explore the pools of uncertainty that still characterise human biology — especially when it comes to applying medical science to human illness. This was something that the Hammersmith in its heyday did uniquely well, and to which Thompson made an enduring contribution.

Preface

Medicine is my lawful wife and literature is my mistress; when I tire of one, I spend the night with the other.

— Anton Chekov

This book is an account of a life motivated by two pursuits: medicine, my profession, and flyfishing, my favourite recreation. Each in their own way has provided me with challenges, enjoyment, and fulfilment. Much of the subject matter is based upon that published previously in *Hammersmith Marathon*[1] and *The Cholesterol Controversy*,[2] both now out of print, and the more recent *Time Spent Fishing*.[3] The resulting narrative records my experiences, mostly medical but some piscatorial, and includes an account of Endo's discovery of statins and their role in proving the lipid hypothesis of atherosclerosis, arguably among the most important advances in cardiovascular research during the latter part of the 20th century.

Life as a medical student at St. Thomas's Hospital in post-war London was probably more akin to what it was like when Somerset Maugham studied there at the end of the 19th century than to what it is now. Taking the daunting examination for Membership of the Royal College of Physicians (MRCP), an essential prerequisite to becoming a consultant physician or a clinical academic, was a bit of a lottery in the late 1950s, when success could depend as much on inspired guesswork as on knowledge. Medical contemporaries conscripted to do military service may recall their time in the Royal Army Medical Corps (RAMC), which in my case included nearly 2 years on secondment to the Ghana Army.

After completing my short service commission in the RAMC in 1963, much of my career was spent at the Royal Postgraduate Medical School

(RPMS) at Hammersmith Hospital, the leading postgraduate teaching centre in Britain and a world-renowned centre of clinical research during the 1950s, 1960s, and 1970s. The Department of Medicine in those days consisted of a group of full-time academic physicians under the successive directorships of John McMichael, Christopher Booth, and Keith Peters, all of whom were later knighted. The highlight of the week was the Staff Round, the equivalent of Grand Rounds in the USA, which took place every Wednesday between 10:15 and 11:30 am and provided up-and-coming young Turks with an opportunity to demonstrate their presentation skills.

Although I trained originally as a gastroenterologist, my career underwent a drastic change of direction following two spells of research in the USA, firstly in Boston and then in Houston. While there, I became increasingly interested in the role of lipids (fats) as the putative cause of atherosclerosis, whereby arteries supplying blood to the heart, brain, and other parts of the body become progressively narrowed by cholesterol-rich plaques, a process known as the lipid hypothesis. To pursue this goal, I resigned my senior lectureship in gastroenterology at the RPMS and instead joined the adjacent Medical Research Council (MRC) Lipid Metabolism Unit directed by Nick Myant. This was at a time when the role of cholesterol in heart disease generated more heat than light among cardiologists, notably Sir John McMichael. Despite or perhaps because of this, the years from 1975 up to 1998, when I retired from the MRC, were the most productive of my career and were spent researching ways and means of preventing or reversing atherosclerosis by lowering blood cholesterol in patients with an inherited tendency to high levels from birth and a predisposition to premature death from heart disease, a disorder known as Familial Hypercholesterolaemia (FH). This included introducing the novel technique of apheresis, involving extracorporeal machine-enabled exchange of cholesterol-free albumin solution for cholesterol-rich plasma, to lower very high cholesterol levels in individuals with homozygous FH, the most extreme form of the disease, and undertaking some of the earliest clinical studies of statins in the UK. Subsequent large, randomised, and controlled trials demonstrated that by lowering cholesterol these drugs arrested atherosclerosis and reduced heart attacks, thus providing conclusive proof of the lipid hypothesis and revolutionising the management of cardiovascular disease worldwide.

For no apparent reason, there seems to be a link between the medical profession and fishing, particularly flyfishing. The prevalence of registered medical practitioners in the UK population in 2015 was 0.43%, whereas 5.7% of the UK-based members of The Flyfishers' Club are medically qualified. Based on this somewhat selective analysis, the proportion of UK doctors that flyfish is more than 10-fold higher than expected — which raises the question, why? For physicians, the attraction may be the fascination of outwitting a wary quarry by employing powers of observation and deduction used to diagnose disease, and for surgeons the application of the manual dexterity acquired in the operating theatre. Whatever the motivation, casting a fly on a Hampshire trout stream or tackling the challenges of salmon fishing in Scotland or Russia provides an ideal escape from the stresses and strains of clinical practice.

The title of this book is a paraphrase of the Chekov quotation cited at the head of the Preface "Medicine is my lawful wife and literature is my mistress." Chekov was a physician and fisherman as well as an author and playwright and another of his sayings was "Time spent fishing does not count towards one's life span." Although there are both physiological and psychological reasons why fishing might be a healthy pastime, there is no conclusive evidence that it increases longevity. That said, a day out on the river with a rod in my hand and hope in my heart undoubtedly has a beneficial effect on me. And should I happen to meet another angler it is possible that he too will be a medic, escaping from the demands of his "lawful wife" and enjoying himself with his piscatorial "mistress."

References

1. Thompson G. *Hammersmith Marathon*. London: Royal Society of Medicine Press, 1999.
2. Thompson G. *The Cholesterol Controversy*. London: Royal Society of Medicine Press, 2008.
3. Thompson G. *Time Spent Fishing*. London: Gilbert Thompson, 2017.

About the Author

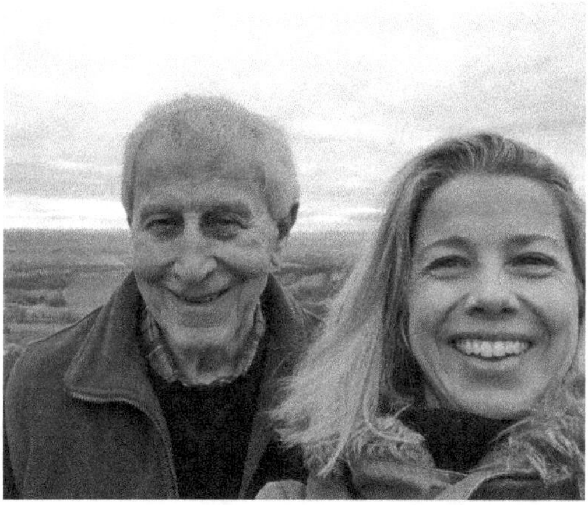

The author and his younger daughter in Yorkshire in 2019.

Gilbert Thompson was born in 1932 and educated at Downside and St. Thomas's Hospital Medical School, London, where he qualified in 1956. After military service, he joined the Royal Postgraduate Medical School, Hammersmith Hospital, London, in 1963 where he worked for most of his career except for periods spent at the Massachusetts General Hospital, Boston, the Methodist Hospital, Houston, and the Royal Victoria Hospital, Montreal, where he was Visiting Professor and recipient of the Lucien Award. He was also a Visiting Professor at the Mayo Clinic in 1997. He led the Medical Research Council Lipoprotein Team and was Professor of Clinical Lipidology at the Royal Postgraduate Medical School, Hammersmith Hospital, where he was Honorary Consultant Physician in charge of the

Lipid Clinic until his retirement in 1998. Currently, he is Emeritus Professor in Clinical Lipidology at the Hammersmith Campus of Imperial College, London.

He is a Past Chairman of the British Atherosclerosis Society, the British Hyperlipidaemia Association, the Forum on Lipids in Clinical Medicine of the Royal Society of Medicine, and the Simon Broome Heart Research Trust. He has been an Associate Editor of the *Journal of Lipid Research* and was the first Editor of *Current Opinion in Lipidology*. He is the author of nine books, 30 chapters, and more than 250 peer-reviewed papers, mainly in the field of lipoprotein metabolism and atherosclerosis.

Acknowledgements

I dedicate this book to the memory of my dear wife Sheila, who died in 2018. We were happily married for 60 years during which she looked after me, ran the house, entertained our guests, accompanied me abroad, and brought up our four children. I could not have survived in the competitive world of academic Medicine nor shared my piscatorial triumphs and disasters without her. My debt to her is immense. In later life, she embarked on a second career as a volunteer at the Royal Botanic Gardens at Kew, her success there being acknowledged by the award of an MBE and the posthumous planting of a tree in her honour.

I am also grateful for the continuing support of my family, friends, and colleagues, and especially to Keith Peters for his perceptive Foreword, written with uniquely authoritative insight into the Hammersmith, apheresis, and clinical research. Finally, I thank Merlin Fox, Koe Shi Ying and S. Balasubramanian, World Scientific Publishing for guiding me through the publication process.

Contents

Foreword v

Preface vii

About the Author xi

Acknowledgements xiii

1. From Fisher's Pond to St. Thomas's 1
2. The Army and the Membership Exam 9
3. Ghana 17
4. From the Hammersmith to Boston 27
5. Texas 37
6. "A Bloody Great Swerve" in Mid-Career 45
7. The Origins of Clinical Lipidology 55
8. Sir John McMichael's Anti-Cholesterol Campaign 65
9. Should Every Cow Carry a Government Health Warning? 75
10. The Discovery of Statins 85
11. Does Lowering Cholesterol Cause Murder and Suicide? 97
12. The Statin Trials Prove the Lipid Hypothesis 105
13. Apheresis — The Cholesterol Take-Away Procedure 117
14. Scotland 129
15. Hazards of Running Marathons 141

16. Exuma 149
17. Russia 159
18. Retirement 169
19. The Expanding Scene of Lipid-Lowering Agents 177
20. Epilogue 187

Index 191

1 From Fisher's Pond to St. Thomas's

India, 1939

To begin at the beginning, I caught my first fish when aged 6 while on holiday with my parents in India. My father, a keen fisherman, was serving there in the British Army and had arranged to spend his leave in Kashmir during the summer of 1939, where there was some excellent trout fishing in those days. Halfway through our trip, he received a telegram informing him that the war had started and ordering him to report back posthaste to his regiment, which was returning to England. So we quickly packed up camp and made our way to Bombay to board a troopship to Marseilles and from there travelled by train to Cherbourg and thence across the Channel by ferry to Southampton. We arrived in England in May 1940 just a couple of weeks before the evacuation of the British Expeditionary Force from Dunkirk. My memory of those days is hazy but I remember our troopship, the converted P&O liner the SS *Strathallan*, passing through the Suez Canal, the last passenger ship to do so before it was closed for the rest of the war; 2 years later the ship was torpedoed and sunk by a German U-boat. I also recall the strange-looking uniforms and helmets of the French soldiers we saw at the railway station in Cherbourg, many of whom were, like us, trying to get to England before it was too late.

Schoolboy

My father spent much of the rest of the war with the 14th Army in the Far East. His absence meant that my early piscatorial education was supervised by my paternal grandfather, a retired general of First World War vintage.

He was an inveterate pipe smoker but real tobacco was hard to come by in those days and instead he smoked an aromatic "heather mixture" which looked and smelled like a smouldering bonfire. He lived in Winchester and during my prep school holidays we would travel by bus to nearby Fisher's Pond and hire a boat for the day. There we would float-fish in the lake with worms for perch and tench but all too often catch eels, which swallowed hook, line, and sinker, retrieval of which sometimes required major surgery. Often our fishing would be interrupted by air raid warnings. Initially we would row ashore every time the sirens sounded but after a while we ignored their wails and fished on regardless. After my father returned from the war in 1946 he introduced my brother and me (Figure 1) to the rudiments of flyfishing during a holiday in Ireland, thereby infecting us both with a lifelong passion for this pastime.

During the spring and summer of 1949, while I was at boarding school, I kept a fishing log. This consisted of a little blue, ink-spotted exercise book in which, under the heading "Downside Fishing Club (Fly)," I meticulously recorded the dates when I had fished, the number and length of trout caught, and the flies responsible. The Comments column included a plaintive "Lost my last Mayfly" and a week later the *cri de coeur* "If only

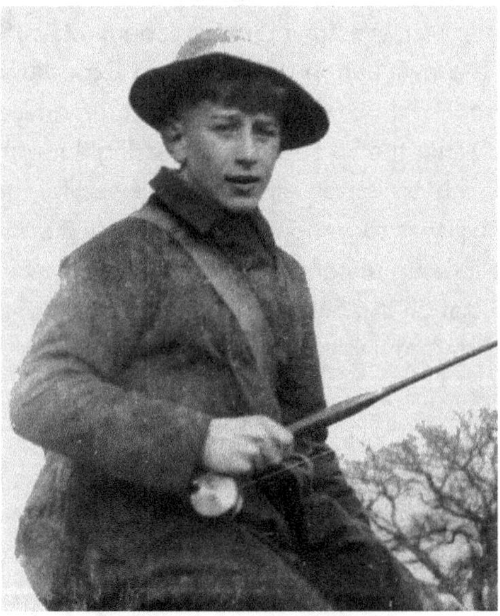

Figure 1. Starting young.

I had a Mayfly." The log ended with a page headed Statistics, which listed the number of fish I caught during the season, their sizes, and which flies caught the most fish. The largest fish weighed ½ lb. These exploits all took place on the little stream that runs through the valley at the bottom of Holcombe Hill in Somerset when I was a pupil at Downside School in nearby Stratton on the Fosse. In retrospect, my fishing log may have been an early indicator of my subsequent interest in collating scientific data.

While I was only 15, I decided that I wanted to become a doctor. I still have the brown-covered scrap book that I kept at the time, filled with anatomical drawings and newspaper cuttings of surgical operations then considered to be state-of-the-art. My choice of career was not viewed with much enthusiasm by my father, partly because he wanted to maintain the strong military tradition in our family and partly because of the financial implications of having to support me for another 6 years after I left school. Both my grandfathers had been soldiers and I had no medical connections. However, my headmaster realised how determined I was and handled my father with a skill that belied his nickname "The Bear," bestowed on him because of his bulk. I still have the letter he wrote to my father which starts "Whilst I still think that Gilbert is not likely to make a successful doctor ..." and my father's note after a subsequent visit to see him that I now was "likely to make a successful doctor." I also still have the copy of Cronin's *The Citadel* given to me as a Christmas present by a supportive female friend of the family in 1948 and inscribed "To Dr. G.T." This book captured my youthful imagination and further encouraged my ambition to become a doctor.

Medical Student

A year or so later I received a letter from St. Thomas's Hospital Medical School informing me that I had obtained a place as a first-year medical student, starting in October 1950. The only snag was that my training was to be financed by a Kitchener Medical Services Scholarship, which entailed a minimum commitment of 5 years in the Royal Army Medical Corps (RAMC) after I qualified. It later transpired that this was a blessing in disguise but it did not seem so to me at the time.

Despite St. Thomas's rather posh reputation, our pre-clinical intake provided an interesting cross-section of society ranging from an Old Etonian

Honourable to a front row forward from Bridgend. A cross-section of male society, to be precise, because there were only 6 women in our intake of 50. My first year was not arduous because I only had zoology and botany to do for my 1st MB, being exempted from taking chemistry and physics after passing both subjects at Higher School Certificate level. This all changed during my second and third years when we started studying anatomy under the critical and sardonic eye of the Professor, a Welsh demagogue whose vivas were both frequent and demanding. We had to memorise a huge amount of detail for these occasions, relying heavily on mnemonics such as "The lingual nerve takes a bloody great swerve around the hyoglossus" to help us. The cadaver I shared with four or five other students was nicknamed "Joe" and we got to know it in intimate detail, especially the penetrating odour of the formalin it exuded. The demands of anatomy were such that there was little time left for physiology, which we were taught by the son of the famous Sir Joseph Barcroft, with the aid of the ubiquitous "smoked drum."

At this stage four of us were sharing a flat in Notting Hill Gate whence we travelled each morning to Lambeth Palace Road in a temperamental Austin 7, which often stalled at Hyde Park Corner and had to be push-started in the midst of the rush hour traffic. Although we had to work hard we managed to maintain the irresponsible image of medical students created by our predecessors over the ages and perpetuated by Charles Dickens. Thus, one Guy Fawkes night, we donned our white dissecting room coats and with brooms at the slope, marched over Lambeth Bridge and along the Embankment to Parliament Square, towing a replica cannon. Once there we fired a salvo of thunder flashes at the Houses of Parliament and then formed up to march back to St. Thomas's. We had just got to Westminster Bridge when a horde of policemen poured out of Canon Row police station and broke up the march. One of our number, nicknamed Foetal Freddie on account of his small stature, was arrested for kicking an officer of the law but was let off later with a caution. The rest of us made it back to base with our cannon intact, delighted with the success of our foray. Needless to say it is definitely not the kind of Guy Fawkes demonstration that would be tolerated nowadays in terrorist-conscious London.

During the Christmas holidays we got temporary jobs at Maiden Lane Goods Depot sorting mail bags. This meant starting work at an unreasonably early hour and was physically demanding due to the coldness of the weather and the weight of the mail bags, which were full of Christmas parcels. There was quite a crowd of us, mainly from Thomas's and the Middlesex Hospital, and our enthusiasm for our work peaked each Friday, which was pay day. Most of what we earned was soon spent on beer and petrol but we enjoyed the novelty of being paid workers. During one winter there was such a prolonged cold spell that we were able to play an impromptu ice hockey match against the Middlesex on the frozen lake in St. James's Park (Figure 2).

Life became easier and more interesting after passing 2nd MB. I moved into a house in Crozier Street just opposite the hospital together with several other medical students, one of whom cooked magnificent curries when hunger and inspiration coincided. Our landlady charged us

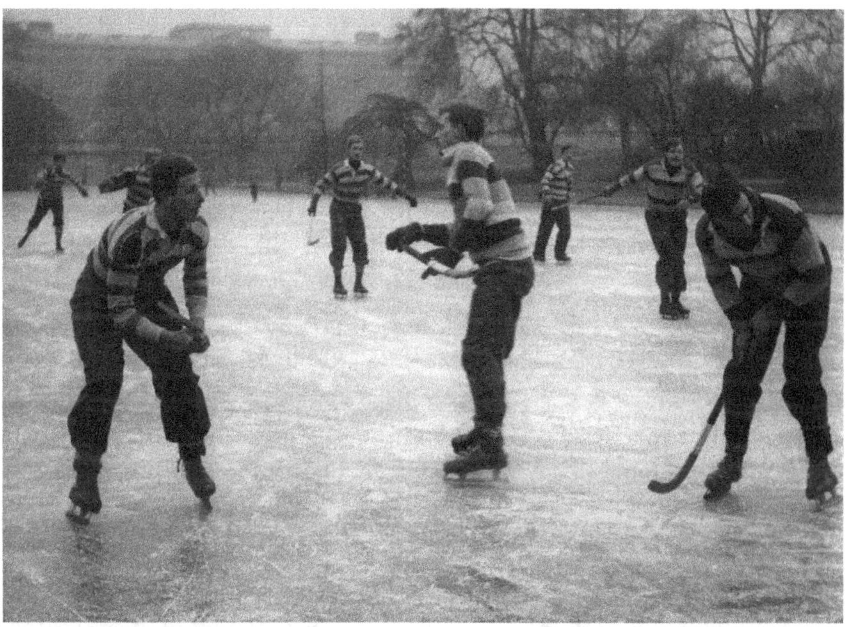

Figure 2. Ice hockey in St. James's Park, with Buckingham Palace in the background.

30 shillings a week, a bargain despite the fact that the only lavatory was outside at the bottom of the garden. To get there necessitated traversing the basement kitchen to get to the backdoor, avoiding treading on the toes of the landlady's large brother or falling over her obese dog in the process. Crozier Street was authentic *Liza of Lambeth*[1] territory but it was subsequently demolished when the area was redeveloped.

Contact with patients in the Casualty department gave us a sense of importance, heightened by being taught to do minor procedures. These included digital blocks, which involved injecting local anaesthetic into the fingers of patients about to be treated for paronychia (nail infection) by avulsion of the nail, and then injecting penicillin into their buttocks, a task made tricky by the large volume and viscosity of the antibiotic suspension. Added zest came from the presence on the wards of nurses, who were called Nightingales in honour of their founder and were selected mainly on the basis of their social background and looks. However, the Sisters were a formidable lot, especially those in charge of the Nurses' Home, and they discriminated between doctors and medical students as unerringly as between frogs and tadpoles.

St. Thomas's was blessed with numerous larger-than-life consultants in those days. One, who specialised in venereology (sexually transmitted diseases), never tired of telling us "He ran a risk, he paid the price" referring to the numerous unfortunates in the department with gonorrhoea or syphilis. Another, a much-loved Welsh cardiologist, had lost the middle two fingers of his right hand during the war and used to hold up this hand with its wide gap between index and little finger saying "Never would have made a gynaecologist, boyo!"

Surgeons too had a sense of humour. On one ward round, the consultant surgeon to whose "firm" we were attached cautioned an attractive female student not to go too near the bed of a recently circumcised man "otherwise he might burst all his stitches." On another occasion, the same surgeon was undertaking a sigmoidoscopy under general anaesthetic. After inserting the stainless steel sigmoidoscope into the patient's rectum, he handed me a rubber bulb resembling a scent spray that was attached to the instrument and told me to compress it. I had no idea of how often or for how long I had to do this so I just kept rhythmically compressing the bulb. After a while the surgeon muttered something about the eye-piece misting up and needing cleaning. As he removed the eye-piece there was a loud report and a brown missile shot out of the sigmoidoscope under considerable pressure and hit the wall of the operating theatre. The surgeon regarded me with a mixture of surprise and respect, saying "Bad luck, my boy, you nearly got me."

During the summer holidays of 1953, I was rock climbing in Llanberis Pass in Snowdonia and was lucky enough to be befriended by and climb with the Cambridge University Mountaineering Club, who were celebrating the return of one of their members, George Band, from the triumphant conquest of Everest. Also climbing there that year were the legendary Joe Brown and Don Whillans, pioneering a series of impossibly difficult routes and taking rock climbing in Britain to new heights. One afternoon, I went from Pen-Y-Gwyrd where I was staying to a shop lower down the Pass to buy some provisions. Behind the counter was a tiny Welsh woman who, after I'd made my purchases, asked me "English are you?" "Yes" I said. "Climbing are you?" "Yes," again. "Well mind you don't end up like the last English climber I served in here. He fell off and came back in a sack!" In actual fact I did fall off while climbing on Cyrn Las in the rain but my running belay cushioned my fall and, taking off my boots, I completed the route successfully in socks and so avoided coming back in a sack.

Our 3 years of clinical training soon passed, a blur of pubs and parties, sports cars, and rugby matches. On the occasion of a Hospitals Cup match versus St. Mary's at the latter's ground, Thomas's supporters like me were bombarded with bags containing a mixture of soot and plaster of Paris and then sprayed with hoses. Once the mixture had set there was no getting it off. I don't remember who won the Cup match, probably St. Mary's, but they certainly won the battle of the supporters.

The highlight of the social year was the annual St. Thomas's Ball at the newly built Royal Festival Hall, an all-night affair. Tickets were expensive but I was determined to get my money's worth and stay awake to the bitter end so took a Dexedrine tablet to ensure I did. However, the mixture of amphetamine and alcohol inspired me to perform the eightsome reel with such vigour that I slipped and cracked my head on the marble floor and was *hors de combat* for the rest of the night.

The time soon came for us to take our finals with all the frantic last minute revision and cramming that this involved. The Professor of Medicine,

Peter Sharpey-Schafer, gave us our results in the local pub, a venue equally suited to celebration and commiseration. I passed and celebrated the fact that I was now a qualified doctor at the ripe old age of 23.

Reference

1. Maugham WS. *Liza of Lambeth,* London: T. Fisher Unwin, 1897.

2 The Army and the Membership Exam

House Officer

The transition from medical student to pre-registration house officer (intern), equivalent nowadays to Foundation Doctor Year 1, was a traumatic process. Responsibility descended upon our shoulders with a sudden and at times overwhelming weight. The hours we worked accentuated the misery of metamorphosis but undoubtedly enabled us to acquire invaluable clinical experience at a rapid rate. Somehow I managed to cope but my natural optimism was quenched by the prospect of 5 years in the army after completing my pre-registration house jobs. This was 3 years more than the 2 years of National Service which I and my contemporaries had to serve as conscripts and I regarded it as a death sentence upon my future medical prospects. How wrong I was.

One experience I'll never forget as a house officer was assisting my boss with the oesophagoscopy of a patient who had developed dysphagia (difficulty in swallowing) a few weeks after swallowing a fish bone. The surgeon inserted and gently slid the stainless steel oesophagoscope (which in those days was rigid but nowadays is flexible) down the sedated patient's oesophagus to ascertain the location and nature of the problem. Suddenly, a torrent of bright red arterial blood erupted up the oesophagus and sprayed over the surgeon and operating theatre. It later transpired that the fish bone had caused a para-oesophageal abscess that had involved and weakened the wall of the adjacent aorta, the largest artery in the body, which the oesophagoscope had inadvertently penetrated.

One other memory, less tragic, was of being rung up by the agent of a famous American film star who was filming in Britain and being asked to arrange for the latter to have his prostate massaged by my boss. I had to explain that this might be a bit tricky as the latter was a neurologist not a urologist!

In the RAMC

In the winter of 1958, now a registered medical practitioner after completing my house jobs, I duly reported to the RAMC barracks at Crookham for basic training (Figure 1). This mainly consisted of being taught to march in step and was a complete waste of time. The sole consolation was the heavy humour employed by non-commissioned officers on the parade ground: "Name? Age? Married or 'appy?" and "Am I hurting you?" "No, Sergeant" "Well I orter be, I'm standing on yer back 'air — get it cut!" After a few weeks of this I passed out (in the military sense) and was sent on a course in military medicine at the RAMC College at Millbank, knowing that if I did

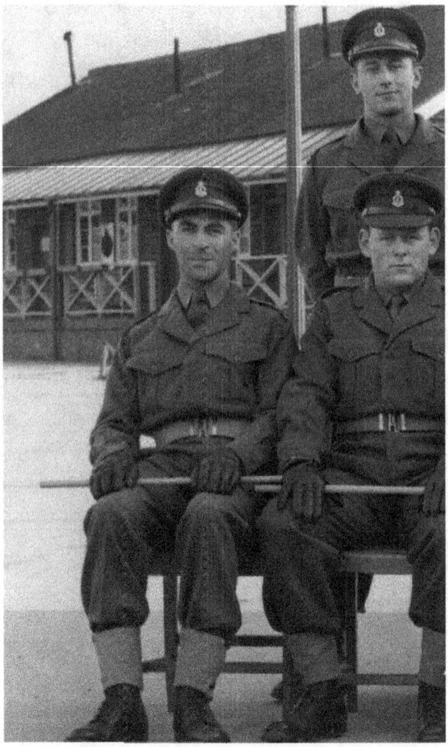

Figure 1. The author (standing) in the RAMC barracks, Crookham.

well I might get the chance to become a Trainee Medical Specialist at the adjacent Queen Alexandra Military Hospital.

I worked hard and, overcoming my natural diffidence, constantly asked questions during lectures so as to get myself noticed. This strategy paid off and I was selected for specialist training, with the immediate objective of gaining membership of the Royal College of Physicians (MRCP), an obligatory step on the pathway to becoming a consultant physician. To its credit, the army gave me the opportunity to attend every worthwhile membership course in London, including one held annually at the London Hospital in Whitechapel. Among the tutors there was Willie Evans, yet another Welsh cardiologist, who decreed that anyone who failed to detect an aortic diastolic murmur (indicative of an incompetent aortic valve) with their stethoscope would have to write out 50 times "I must listen to diastole." Another was Donald Hunter, who insisted that sieving a patient's stools through one's girlfriend's black nylon stockings was the best method of detecting the white, pin-sized head of a tapeworm that proved treatment of the latter had been successful. Tapeworm infestation in London in those days was quite common in fashion models, the unintended consequence of a liking for steak tartare.

In the summer of 1958, I married a lovely Dutch girl to whom I'd been engaged for several years while I was a medical student. I invited several Thomas's friends over to Holland and a memorable stag party ensued the night before the wedding. Unfortunately, I was barely able to stand the next day in church and I leaned heavily upon the arm of my new bride coming down the aisle. The damage had been done by a life-sized glass Wellington boot which was filled and refilled with a mixture of mainly beer and genever (Dutch gin). The boot circulated from hand to hand as the evening wore on but inevitably each round ended with my having to finish off what was left in the toe of the boot. I drank nothing but water during the wedding dinner the next day, much to the disgust of my father-in-law who had laid on some fine wines for the occasion. My friends were in no better shape except for one who had previously been an alcoholic but who had recently taken the pledge. The current custom of separating by several days the stag party and the wedding has much to commend it.

One of the ushers at our wedding was about to start a house job at Hammersmith Hospital, known colloquially as The Hammersmith and regarded as the mecca of clinical research in Britain. He invited me to pay him a visit when I got back from my honeymoon. I duly did so and he brought me along to the weekly Department of Medicine Staff Round, which in those days took place in a small lecture theatre at the far end of the very long hospital corridor. The room was packed with medical staff and postgraduates who were eager spectators at what seemed like a verbal free-for-all among the consultants standing at the front. My friend pointed out several whose names were legendary at that time, including the endocrinologist Russell Fraser, the nephrologist Malcolm Milne, the rheumatologist Eric Bywaters, and the hepatologist Sheila Sherlock. The atmosphere was informal and argumentative and I resolved there and then that this was the place for me — if I could get in. First, however, I had to get my MRCP and survive the years I still had to serve in the RAMC.

The MRCP Exam

As one might expect, the membership exam has changed considerably during the past 60 years. In those days it consisted of two written papers, clinical exams, a pathology viva, and a final viva, all within the period of a month. All candidates took the written papers and the clinicals and the minority who passed both were invited to the pathology viva. This resulted in further fall out and the lucky few who survived were invited to the final viva at the College, which was then situated in Pall Mall East near Trafalgar Square.

The papers weren't too difficult and, happily for me, included a question on hydatid disease (a parasitic disease acquired from contact with dog faeces), which had been covered in detail on the RAMC College course. My clinicals were at Guy's and while I waited, an old school friend and RAMC colleague told me all about the case he'd just seen. When my turn came I immediately realised that mine was the same case. I rattled off all the physical signs to the examiner, ending with the gilt on the gingerbread, namely that the patient had secondary optic atrophy. The examiner, an elderly Scottish chest physician, nodded sagely but then unexpectedly inquired which eye was the worst affected. My friend had not told me the answer to this question so, feigning a confidence I did not feel, I said "Right eye, Sir." The examiner slowly got to his feet, picked up an ophthalmoscope and peered first in one eye and then in the other. Having done so, he sat down slowly, looked up at me and said "Yes, I agree."

A letter in the post the following week stated, "If you will attend at the Examination Hall in Queen Square … your examination will be continued." I got a similar letter after the Path viva inviting me to the Royal College of Physicians for the final viva. Less than 40 of the original 300 candidates got as far as a final viva although most of those that did so would pass. However, the unlucky few who failed the final viva would have to start again from scratch, just like the game Snakes and Ladders.

The invitation was for 2 pm but, arriving early, I killed time by walking endlessly around the precinct in Pall Mall where the College was situated. Eventually the time came to enter the hallowed portals whereupon I was asked to wait in the library before being ushered into the Censors' Room. This contained a long table at the far end of which sat the President on a raised dais, flanked by three examiners on either side, while I sat alone at the near end. Each examiner in turn asked me a question which I was able to cope with reasonably well until it came to the last examiner, an elderly man who I later discovered was a paediatrician. He asked me to name the commonest cause of acute laryngeal spasm in children in Casualty. "Inhalation of a peanut" I answered confidently but it was not the answer he wanted. He became increasingly tetchy as I went through the entire litany of nuts and a long pause then ensued, during which I could see the exam slipping out of my grasp. Suddenly inspiration came as the silent voice of my guardian angel whispered the magic letters "ATS." "Anaphylactic reaction to anti-tetanus serum, Sir" I blurted out. Although it still wasn't the answer he wanted, which was laryngismus stridulus (spasmodic croup due to rickets) I later discovered, the other examiners seemed impressed with my improvisation and I was ushered into the adjacent office to await their decision. Eventually a hand came through the door with an envelope which the secretary took and opened. She read it and then looked at me and said, "You've passed; please make out a cheque for £31-10 shillings." My request to post-date my cheque was curtly refused but nothing could dim the overwhelming sense of achievement and elation that I felt at that moment.

This all took place in the summer of 1959 when my pregnant wife and I were living in a top floor flat off the Old Brompton Road. Our first child was born the following month in The Lambeth Hospital, just across the river from Millbank, where my wife was under the care of a formidable but kindly female obstetrician. There is a story, probably apocryphal, that on one of her ward rounds she stopped beside the cot of a recent delivery and asked the mother whether her beautiful baby had inherited its red hair from its father. "I don't know, Ma'am" she replied, "he never took his hat off."

My military superiors were pleased albeit somewhat surprised by my success in the MRCP and looked around for a suitable posting for me. I suggested a military hospital in Germany, just over the border from my Dutch in-laws, but there was no vacancy for anyone so junior. Instead, I was given two options: the first was Cowglen, near Glasgow. "Don't advise you to go there, old boy, the last chap there shot himself. How about Accra, Ghana? Used to be called the Gold Coast or White Man's Grave, you know. But don't let that put you off, things have improved since those days." So I volunteered to be seconded to the Ghana Army as the medical specialist at the Military Hospital, Accra, a few months after getting my membership and a couple of years after Ghana had become the first African colony to gain independence from Britain.

Locum Medical Officer to the Horse Guards

There was a gap of a few months before I was due to take up my new post, during which I successfully took the exam for the Diploma of Tropical Medicine and Hygiene (DTM&H), a subject in which the RAMC College specialised. Together with a colleague, who later became a renowned nephrologist, I also undertook duty as locum medical officer at the Horse Guards Barracks in Knightsbridge. When we reported for duty at the officers' mess the adjutant, without removing his boots from the mantelpiece over the fireplace turned to look at us and observing our dark suits and bowler hats, regulation uniform in London, enquired languidly "Are you the bailiffs?"

While at Knightsbridge I was called upon to sew up the mouth of a bandsman who played the French horn and had been bitten by his horse. Otherwise there was not a lot to do apart from accompanying the senior medical officer to do sick parades at the Home Postal Depot, which was located at Wormwood Scrubs between the prison and Hammersmith Hospital. Despite the fact that it was winter all those reporting sick, whatever the reason, were required to stand stark naked in the shower area.

The surgeon colonel then ordered each man to bend over as he passed behind them and inspected them for piles. All those without this complaint were passed fit for duty.

Back at Knightsbridge Barracks, I heard this same officer give the shortest and most powerful lecture on "preventive medicine" that I have ever heard. He was lecturing the new intake of recruits on what he regarded as the perils of homosexuality, believing that their youth and Horse Guards uniforms made them attractive prey for predatory males; his allegorical description of the act of sodomy was unforgettable but unrepeatable in this age of political correctness.

3 Ghana

Voyage to West Africa

In December 1959, my wife and I and our 3-month-old daughter set off from London for Liverpool along the brand new M1 in my brand new Peerless, a fibre-glass-bodied coupe version of a Triumph TR3. In retrospect, this was a thoroughly unsuitable vehicle to take to Ghana because of its low ground clearance but there were tax advantages in doing so. On arrival at the Liverpool docks, we boarded the SS *Apapa* bound for the Ghanaian port of Takoradi, with brief stops at Bathurst, Gambia, and Freetown, Sierra Leone, *en route*. First, however, we had to survive the Bay of Biscay, which lived up to its reputation. Severe seasickness kept us both horizontal for several days, which made feeding the baby, who was unaffected, remarkably difficult. I had to crawl over to the cot and blindly probe around with the bottle until the crying stopped. Feeling better when we got to Freetown, we went ashore leaving the baby on board in the care of a friend. However, we overstayed our welcome at the Club and literally nearly missed the boat. It took a hair-raising taxi drive downhill in response to the ship's siren and a frantic rush across the gangplank to get back on board before the ship departed with our daughter.

On arrival at Takoradi our car was unloaded but could not be moved off the quay because the hand brake was jammed. I got under the car to try to find the problem but failed to do so and emerged half an hour later pouring sweat and covered in oil and dust. My wife proved that she was more than just a pretty face by somehow releasing the hand brake without getting dirty. We then set off along the coast towards Accra, 100 miles to the east, trying to avoid the occasional snake crossing the road ahead of us.

Military Hospital, Accra

The Military Hospital, known as No. 37, was on the outskirts of Accra and had been built during the Second World War. We lived initially in Hospital House, a spacious but far from modern abode that had previously been an officers' mess. We were looked after by a cook, a steward and a "boy" who washed and ironed our clothes daily. The climate was hot and humid and it didn't take us long to realise that the temperature inside Hospital House was much the same as it was outside. The house had a spacious front drive and on one occasion my wife was pushing a pram containing our infant daughter along it when a large spitting cobra crossed her path, causing her considerable alarm but no harm. Later, we moved to a smaller house near the airport which was far cooler and better suited to family life. The main nuisance there was flying ants, which carpeted the veranda several inches deep with their bodies after their annual exodus from the termite hills in our back garden. The locals said they were very tasty but we didn't put this to the test.

Accra is situated close to the intersection of 0° longitude with the Equator and the noonday sun there is nearly vertical all the year round. This was reflected in our uniforms which consisted of open-necked safari-style jackets, shorts, and long socks. The temperature dropped slightly in the rainy season but this was offset by an increase in humidity.

The medical staff of No. 37 comprised a surgeon, a physician (myself), an anaesthetist, a radiologist, an obstetrician, a paediatrician, and 3 medical officers. The paediatrician was Ghanaian but the rest of us were British. Our main task was to look after the Ghana Army and the Police but we were also expected to provide medical cover for local politicians and diplomats as well as visiting dignitaries. On one occasion a small Ghanaian, dressed in traditional garb, came to the front door of our house. My wife, thinking he must be a friend of one of the servants, directed him round to the back of the house. He soon reappeared, however, accompanied by our embarrassed cook who announced that he was the Minister of Health and in need of my advice. Fortunately, like most Ghanaians, the Minister had a good sense of humour.

Labadi Beach was nearby and provided an opportunity to swim and body surf on gentle Atlantic rollers (Figure 1). If one wished to get away from

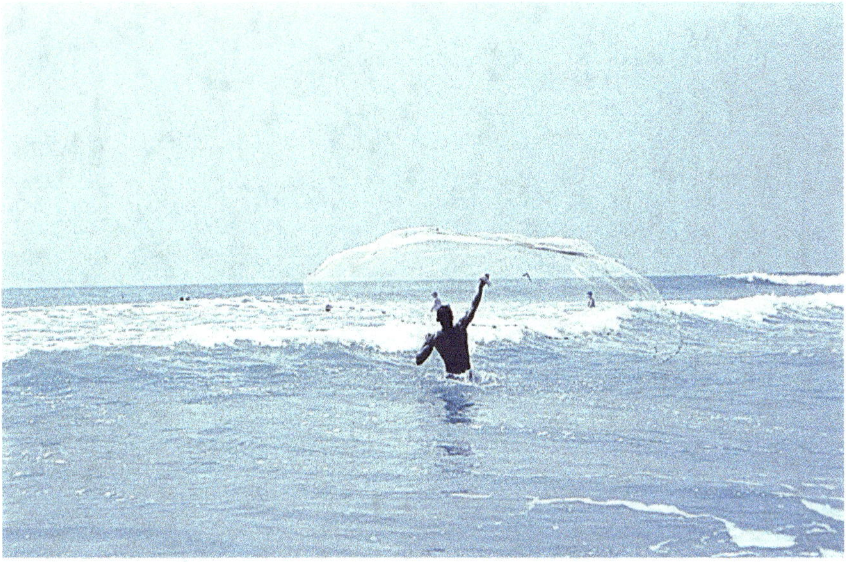

Figure 1. Fishing with a throw net off Labadi Beach, Accra.

Accra, the Army had a guest house at Winneba which could be booked for weekends and which had its own salt water swimming pool (Figure 2). In the evenings, one sat on the stoep with a cold beer and watched the sun go down over Africa, wearing protective knee-length boots to avoid being bitten by mosquitoes. At night, we slept under mosquito netting and the whole family religiously took a daily dose of Paludrine, an anti-malarial to which in those days the local malarial parasites had not yet become resistant.

Among the notables who stopped over in Accra at that time were Dag Hammarskjöld, Secretary General of the United Nations, who died soon after when his plane crashed in what is now Zambia, and Harold MacMillan, the British Prime Minister who was on his "Wind of Change" tour of Africa. The foremost local politician was the recently elected President Kwame Nkrumah, a charming man who I saw on a couple of occasions for his annual health check. I was also required to look after the diplomats of several embassies, including the American and Israeli embassies and the British High Commission. Sometimes this needed diplomacy rather than medical skills, especially when alcohol was involved. Another occasional task was to treat US aircrew landing in Accra, some of whom arrived at the

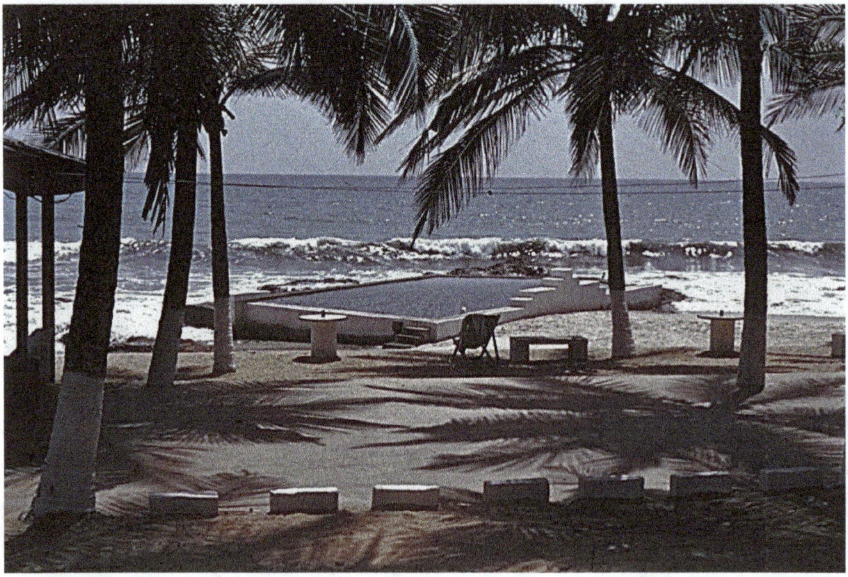

Figure 2. Swimming pool at Winneba.

hospital with an intravenous cortisone drip in one arm and an antibiotic drip in the other. Most of them turned out to have malaria, which they had acquired in the Republic of Congo while ferrying UN soldiers there during the crisis that arose after it became independent from Belgium in 1960, and which soon responded to chloroquine.

The commonest acute medical problems among the Ghanaian soldiers and policemen and their families were malaria, measles and in the Northern Territories (NTs), meningococcal meningitis. One could make a provisional diagnosis of malaria with reasonable certainty at 50 yards if one saw an African walking towards Casualty wearing an overcoat despite the heat. There was also the occasional case of small pox, which thankfully is now extinct. Chronic disorders included pulmonary tuberculosis (TB), leprosy, and parasitic diseases such as schistosomiasis, onchocerciasis (river blindness), and guinea worm. Treatment of the latter necessitated slowly winding out the yard long worm from the ankle onto a matchstick. Great care was needed to prevent breakage of the worm, which resulted in severe inflammation of the whole leg if it occurred.

On one occasion a soldier came to see me complaining that "Sir, I no get power." I deduced that this meant he was impotent and as he seemed fit enough otherwise, I concluded it could be psychogenic. Knowing that his next stop would probably be a Ju-Ju man (witch doctor) I decided to try to pre-empt this with some placebo therapy in the form of an injection of sterile isotonic saline into his buttock, which I assured him would do the trick. He came back beaming a week later saying "Thank you, Sir, I now get plenty power, my wife very happy!"

Abnormal Haemoglobins and Malaria

About one-third of the population of Ghana carries a copy of the genes for the abnormal haemoglobins S or C, either in combination with the normal haemoglobin A or with themselves or with each other. Genes consist of paired alleles, with one allele derived from each parent. Two-thirds of Ghanaians have the normal haemoglobin AA pattern, the remainder have either the AS, AC, SC, SS, or CC pattern in descending order of frequency. About 5 years previously, research workers in Accra had demonstrated a protective effect against falciparum malaria of heterozygous inheritance of haemoglobin S (i.e. AS). Falciparum malaria (also known as malignant tertian) was endemic in West Africa and a major contributor to infant mortality. This was due to its predilection to cause cerebral malaria and acute haemolytic anaemia, manifested by fits and haemoglobinuria (black water fever), respectively, both often fatal. The research had shown that children with the AS pattern (sickle cell trait) were less likely to develop these complications than those with the normal AA pattern. This protective effect of haemoglobin S was thought to explain its spread across Africa at the expense of haemoglobin A, despite the fact that the much rarer homozygous inheritance of haemoglobin S (i.e. SS) resulted in sickle cell disease and was usually fatal. This trade-off is termed balanced polymorphism by geneticists.

I became particularly interested in haemoglobin C, which was especially prevalent in the NTs, from where a high proportion of the policemen in Accra originated (Figure 3). Haemoglobin C was not as common as haemoglobin S and had a more localised distribution, suggesting that the mutation responsible was of more recent origin. Unlike haemoglobin S,

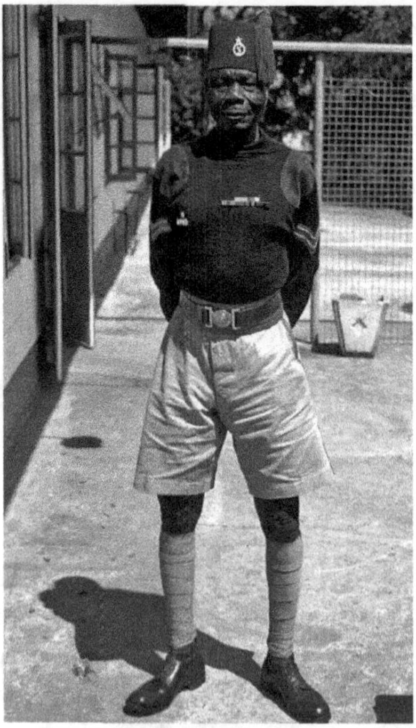

Figure 3. Policeman from the Northern Territories of Ghana.

homozygosity for haemoglobin C (i.e. CC) is a relatively benign disorder so that any protective effect against falciparum malaria of heterozygous inheritance of haemoglobin C (i.e. AC) need not be as great to maintain balanced polymorphism as that conferred by the sickle cell trait. However, a study conducted previously in Ghana had failed to find any evidence of a protective effect of haemoglobin C against malaria.[1]

I decided to test this hypothesis myself and began by constructing a plastic tank for undertaking paper electrophoresis, which would enable me to distinguish between haemoglobin A, S, and C in blood samples. I managed to install an air conditioner in my little "lab" to cool the apparatus and perhaps because of this my wife, who had studied Chemistry at Leiden University before we married, readily volunteered to help! Since policemen, unlike the army, did not receive anti-malarial prophylaxis, we determined the haemoglobin pattern (phenotype) of all policemen and their children who presented with a fever and examined thick films of their blood under the microscope to determine the density of *Plasmodium falciparum* parasites, an index of the severity of malarial infection. The results suggested that not only children with the sickle cell trait but also those carrying haemoglobin C developed less severe parasitaemia than normal individuals with solely haemoglobin A in their red cells, the first time that this had ever been reported.[2] The validity of this hypothesis has since been confirmed by the findings of several large epidemiological studies in Mali, Burkino Faso, and Ghana,[3–5] including one published in *Nature* [6] which concluded that in the absence of malaria control, the protective effect of haemoglobin C would eventually lead to its replacing haemoglobin S in West Africa by a process of natural selection.

A Christmas Turkey

Life in Ghana had its share of both comedy and tragedy. A few weeks before Christmas one of my patients presented me with a live turkey, its wattled head protruding from the top of a brown paper bag tied up with string. I took it home and handed it over to Elijah, our cook cum steward, to fatten up for Christmas. On Christmas Eve he approached me with a request for a bottle of whisky which he said would soften up the turkey and make it more edible. An hour or so later we heard shouts and found the inebriated turkey being chased around the garden by an intoxicated Elijah, who was swiping wildly at the bird with his machete. Eventually, the *coup de grace* was administered and the turkey was served up the next day by a hungover cook. Despite the whisky it was pretty tough to eat.

Elijah was a Nigerian from Port Harcourt and he came to us with a reputation for deterring thieves, based upon the probably apocryphal story that when working for a previous employer he had seen an arm coming in through a window one night and had promptly cut it off with his machete. True or not, we never got burgled.

A Question of Rabies

Much of the emergency work involved treating children who had been brought to Casualty. One of these was an infant with convulsions who died soon after being seen by the medical officer on call. The latter phoned me later that day to say that the parents had subsequently revealed that their infant had been bitten previously by a dog. The medical officer was worried about the possibility of rabies, especially since the baby had salivated over his hands which he'd scratched doing some gardening the previous day. Further enquiries revealed that the baby's body had been taken to its family's village for burial.

I hastily recruited the help of the quartermaster sergeant, who luckily happened to come from the same village, and we set off by car in the gathering darkness. Eventually we reached the village, which had no electricity, to discover that the baby had been buried already and that the wake was in progress. Libations of Akpeteshie, a locally distilled spirit, were being poured onto the grave and down mourners' throats, the scene being lit by the flickering flames of torches. To his great credit the quartermaster managed to get the body disinterred without causing a riot and we took it back to Accra that night. The baby's brain was sent to Lagos, Nigeria for diagnosis and the medical officer was started on a course of injections of anti-rabies vaccine while awaiting the outcome. Happily, the brain histology was negative and the spectre of rabies was exorcised, much to the relief of all concerned.

The Return Home

After nearly 2 years in Accra the climate started to take its toll and we longed for the bracing feel of autumn in England. By now there were four of us in the family and, having completed my tour of duty, I arranged for us to return home by air. We took a KLM flight from Lagos to Amsterdam, feasting our eyes on snow-covered peaks as we crossed the Alps. The plane, one of the subsequently ill-fated Lockheed Electras, eventually got us to fog-bound Holland. After a brief holiday with my Dutch in-laws, we returned to England where I was due to take up my new post as a junior medical specialist at the Queen Alexandra Military Hospital, Millbank.

Before leaving Ghana I had submitted an abstract of my research on malaria and haemoglobins S and C for presentation at a scientific meeting to be held at the Royal College of Physicians in London and organised by Chris Booth. The abstract was accepted and my wife typed out the tables of data on a portable typewriter, which I then photographed on the sitting room floor. Despite my crude slides, the paper was well received and I was complimented afterwards by John McMichael, Professor of Medicine at the Hammersmith. He was impressed that I had managed to undertake research under such adverse circumstances and told me to get in touch with him if I ever wanted a job because the conditions for research at the Hammersmith were not too different!

MD Thesis

My job at Millbank was not arduous and gave me the opportunity to write up the work I had done in Ghana for submission as an MD thesis. This was then typed out laboriously by my wife on her portable typewriter, which was no mean task since the thesis was over 200 pages long and the University of London required 4 bound copies to be submitted. Apart from the data on malaria and haemoglobins S and C, it also included observations I had made on Ghanaian soldiers returning from serving with the United Nations in what had previously been the Belgian Congo. They flew back from Leopoldville (now Kinshasa) in unpressurised Hastings transport planes and a few of them had sustained splenic infarcts (acute blockage of the blood supply to the spleen, often requiring splenectomy) during the flights; all were later shown to have either the sickle cell trait or haemoglobin SC disease. I proposed that the splenic infarcts were due to their haemoglobin S-containing red cells undergoing sickling (deformation) as a result of hypoxia during the flights, which were at an altitude of about 10,000 feet.[7] Although the decrease in the oxygen saturation of red cells that occurred at this altitude was too slight to have adverse effects in normal individuals with the haemoglobin AA pattern it appeared to be enough to induce sickling in some of those with >40% haemoglobin S in their red cells. Had the aircraft been pressurised to 8,000 feet as happens on civil aircraft, this problem would probably not have occurred.

An association between the sickle cell trait and splenic infarcts had been described previously but it was a controversial topic in the eyes of many haematologists, including the External Examiner of my MD thesis. He wanted more data including X-ray evidence before he would accept the diagnosis of splenic infarction. I eventually managed to get the relevant X-rays from a colleague of mine who was still serving in Accra but incorporating it into the thesis meant that much of it had to be re-typed by my long-suffering wife and all four copies then re-bound. However, thanks to her help and the support I got from Hermann Lehman at St. Bartholomew's Hospital, who acted as my supervisor, the revised thesis was eventually accepted and I got my MD.[8]

References

1. Edington GM, Laing WN. Relationship between haemoglobins C and S and malaria in Ghana. *Br Med J* 1957;**ii**:143–5.
2. Thompson GR. Significance of haemoglobins S and C in Ghana. *Br Med J* 1962;**i**:682–5.
3. Agarwal A, Guindo A, Cissoko Y *et al.* Hemoglobin C associated with protection from severe malaria in the Dogon of Mali, a West African population with a low prevalence of haemoglobin S. *Blood* 2000;**96**:2358–62.
4. Rihet P, Flori L, Tall F *et al.* Hemoglobin C is associated with reduced *Plasmodium falciparum* parasitemia and low risk of mild malaria attack. *Hum Mol Genet* 2004;**13**:1–6.
5. Mockenhaupt FP, Ehrhardt S, Cramer JP *et al.* Hemoglobin C and resistance to severe malaria in Ghanaian children. *J Infect Dis* 2004;**190**:1006–9.
6. Modiano D, Luoni G, Sirima BS *et al.* Hemoglobin C protects against clinical Plasmodium falciparum malaria. *Nature* 2001;**414**:305–8.
7. Thompson GR. Malaria and stress in relation to haemoglobins S and C. *Br Med J* 1963;**ii**:976–8.
8. Thompson GR. *The significance of haemoglobins S and C in Ghana.* MD Thesis, University of London, 1963.

4 From the Hammersmith to Boston

The Hammersmith

My chief ambition was to get a job at the Hammersmith after leaving the army and, in view of my recent experiences in Ghana, I hoped there might be an opportunity to pursue a career in haematology. However, this specialty was almost entirely laboratory orientated at the Hammersmith, under the direction of Professor John Dacie, whereas I was more interested in clinical work. It so happened that haematological patients were admitted under the care of the gastroenterologist, Chris Booth, who had a vacancy for a registrar coming up at around the time when I was due to complete my 5 years short service commission in the RAMC. I applied and was duly invited for interview. This proved relatively straightforward until it was the turn of Moran Campbell, a dynamic and extrovert chest physician, to question me. We disagreed on the impact of pH on the oxygen dissociation curve of haemoglobin (the relationship between its oxygen content and the partial pressure of oxygen) and although in retrospect he was probably correct, at the time I thought I was and stood my ground. My argumentative attitude did me no harm in the eyes of Professor McMichael and the other members of the selection committee and I was offered a job as medical registrar, starting on January 1, 1963.

The political climate at the start of 1963 was fraught. The Cuban missile crisis had just taken place and had caused my wife and I to stock up the cellar of our house in London with non-perishable items of food and bottles of water in case our children survived the anticipated nuclear war longer than we did. Thankfully, this was averted by President Kennedy successfully challenging Khrushchev but his popular triumph was abruptly cut short by his tragic assassination in Dallas in November. Winter at the

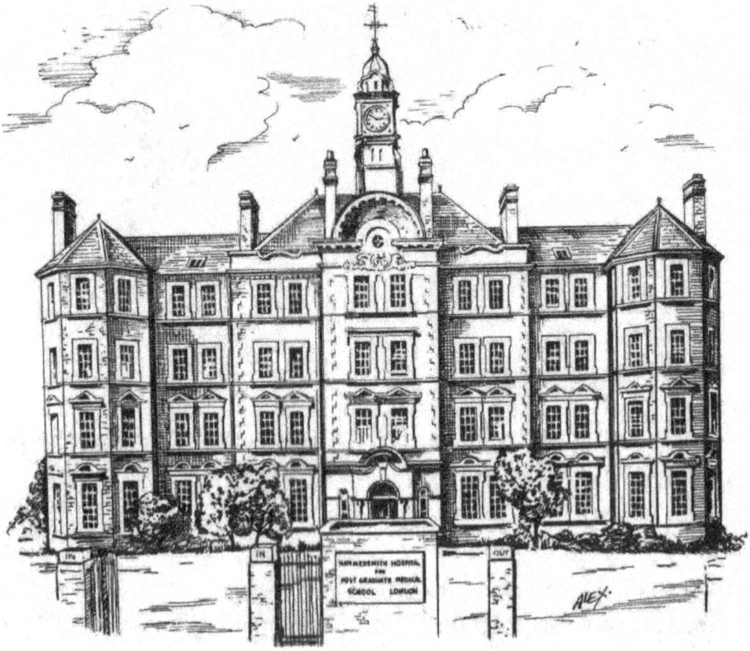

Figure 1. Hammersmith Hospital and Postgraduate Medical School in the 1960s (from a Christmas card sold by the Friends of Hammersmith Hospital).

start of the year in Britain was also fraught and the temperature inside the hospital was similar to that outside. Built in 1905, the building was not old enough to be architecturally distinguished nor recent enough to be modern (Figure 1). However, it was marginally less forbidding than the adjacent prison. Both institutions faced DuCane Road in West London and backed onto the large, grassy expanse of Wormwood Scrubs, after which the prison was named.

The Gastroenterology Unit

The gastroenterology laboratory consisted of a room without a view in a glorified Nissen Hut in the Lower Medical Corridor. I was allocated a space at the lab table and spent several months twiddling my thumbs, wondering what to do. The house physician, the late Graham Neale, was exceptionally

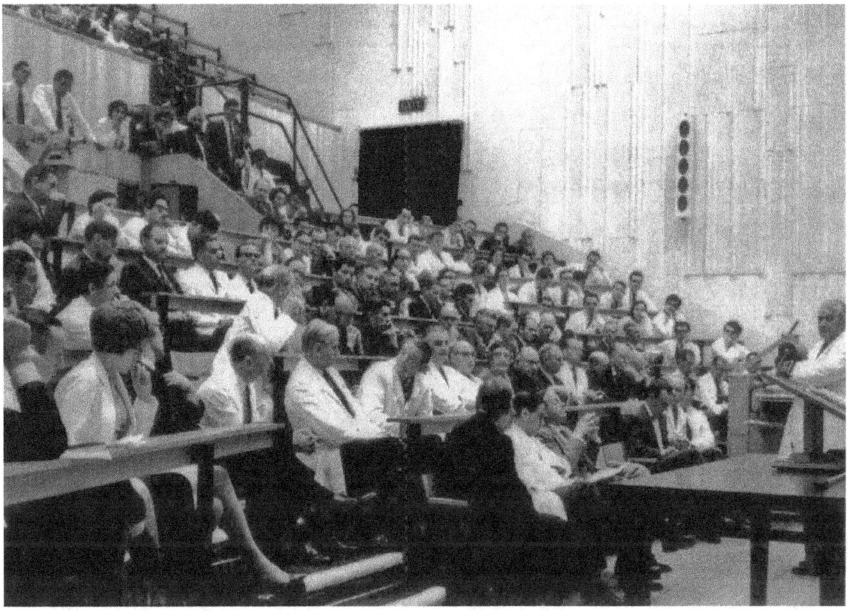

Figure 2. The Hammersmith Staff Round in 1966, chaired by Professor McMichael.

competent and had no need for my advice on the wards. Clinically, I felt redundant and there was no obvious research niche into which I could fit. That is to say, not until we admitted a patient called Ivy and I had to present her case on the Staff Round.

Presenting a case on the Staff Round was quite an ordeal both for the presenter, usually a registrar (resident), and for the consultant in charge of the patient (Figure 2). Within the 10 minutes allotted to presenting the case one had to bring out the salient points of what was often a complex clinical problem, sometimes stretching over many years. In those days the presenter had the details of the case history and findings typed on a white card and projected via an industrial sized epidiascope, interpolated with ECG tracings, X-rays, and histology slides. Nowadays, this is all done with the aid of a computer and PowerPoint. Afterwards, there was 15 minutes for discussion of the case, open to all. No microphones were allowed, which taught one the importance of an audible delivery, a useful asset for later life on the lecture circuit.

Vitamin D Deficiency

To return to Ivy, she was an elderly woman living alone in squalid circumstances in West London who had developed severe osteomalacia (adult rickets) as a consequence of vitamin D deficiency. We concluded that this was secondary to steatorrhoea (malabsorption of fatty substances) caused by a stricture of the terminal part of the small intestine.[1] This resulted in an inability to reabsorb bile acids, which are needed for fat absorption. Proof that she did indeed malabsorb vitamin D, a fat soluble compound, was obtained by demonstrating increased excretion of radioactivity in her stools after an oral dose of tritium-labelled vitamin D, a novel investigation at the time. Following prolonged treatment with injections of vitamin D, her osteomalacia gradually healed and she was able to walk again 15 months later.

Our ability to measure vitamin D absorption for the first time in humans enabled us to investigate various other gastrointestinal disorders known to be associated with bone disease.[2] This included patients with the post-gastrectomy syndrome in whom vitamin D deficiency was common.[3] However, we showed that in most instances their absorption of vitamin D was normal, suggesting that poor diet and inadequate sunlight were the main cause of their osteomalacia.[4] Unlike Ivy, they could be treated with oral supplements of vitamin D.

Measuring faecal fat excretion involved collecting 3 days' worth of stools in large tins that were then stored in a fume cupboard prior to analysis. In warm weather, the gas pressure within the tins built up and periodically their lids blew off with predictably unpleasant consequences. I began to see what McMichael had meant about the conditions for doing research at the Hammersmith being similar to Ghana.

I sent in an abstract of our research on vitamin D absorption for presentation at a meeting of the Medical Research Society (MRS) at the Royal Free Hospital, chaired by Professor Sheila Sherlock. This was my first experience of the MRS which insisted that papers should be spoken not read. Chris Booth rehearsed me time after time until I knew my presentation by heart. When my turn came I stepped up to the podium and said "First slide please." A slide appeared but it was the summary slide. All my pent-up adrenaline was released and I shouted "Not the last slide, the first!"

The projector went off and this was followed by the unmistakeable clatter of slides falling onto the floor. One of my colleagues rushed back to the projection room to try to put the slides back in their correct sequence while I fumed and Sheila Sherlock looked increasingly impatient. I eventually got started again but inevitably my presentation was something of an anticlimax. Subsequently, however, our findings were published in the prestigious American *Journal of Clinical Investigation*,[2] which impressed the Hammersmith hierarchy.

My work on vitamin D put me in touch with Philippe Bordier, a charismatic French physician, whose main research interest was the pathophysiology of bone. Chris Booth and I first met him in Cambridge at a meeting of the Bone and Tooth Club, an occasion notable for the fact that in order to get there in time I overtook a police car at more than 100 mph in my Peerless, which I'd brought back from Ghana. There were no speed limits in those days but, even so, the policemen looked slightly startled as we sped past them.

Philippe worked at the Hôpital Lariboisiere in Paris and Chris arranged for me to go over there to work with him for a few weeks. He met me at the Gare du Nord in his MG, which he'd parked in a one way street. He decided with Gallic logic that it was legal to reverse down this street but this was disputed by the gendarme directing traffic from his pedestal on a nearby roundabout who blew his whistle and shouted in French "Hey you, do you think you're in a circus?" whereupon Philippe retorted as we sped away "If I'm in the circus, you must be the clown!" I became firm friends with him and his wife Michelle and we combined work and pleasure with equal success. Later they both acquired Mini Coopers and used to race each other home from the centre of Paris to their beautiful chateau at Le Mée. Tragically Philippe died when he was only 50.

The Mass General Hospital, Boston

After 2 years at the Hammersmith I was appointed senior registrar in gastroenterology. In those days a BTA (Been To America) was an important addition to one's CV so I applied for a Medical Research Council (MRC) Travelling Fellowship to go and work with Kurt Isselbacher at the Massachusetts General Hospital (MGH) in Boston, known colloquially as

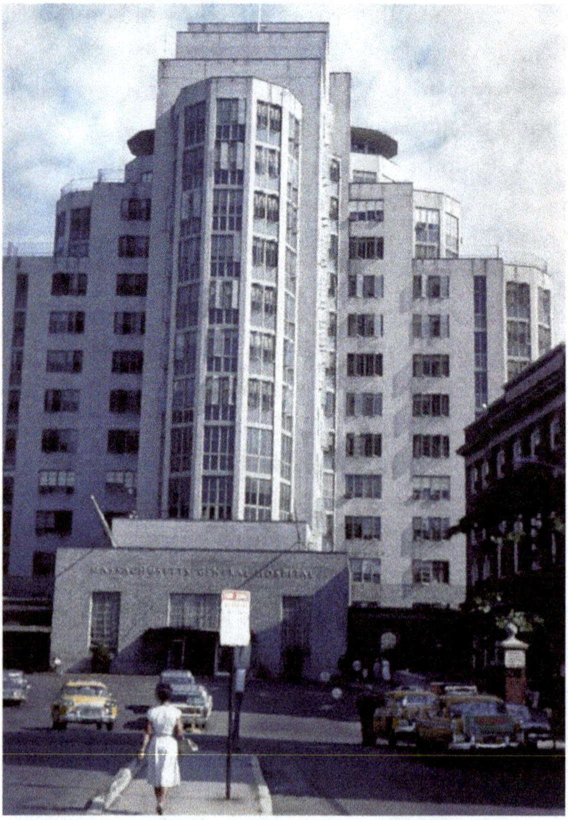

Figure 3. The Massachusetts General Hospital in 1967.

the Mass General (Figure 3). Thanks to John McMichael's and Chris Booth's backing I was successful and was appointed a Research Fellow at Harvard Medical School, with which the MGH was affiliated. The latter was regarded as the top teaching hospital in the USA and competition for internships was fierce. Among the interns, while I was there, were Joe Goldstein and Mike Brown, both future Nobel Prize winners. Interns used to present cases at Grand Rounds in the revered Ether Dome, where the atmosphere was more formal than at the Staff Round and the subsequent discussion was often a commentary by an invited expert, in contrast to the free for all approach at the Hammersmith.

Under the supervision of Kurt Isselbacher my work at the MGH was directed towards investigating factors influencing vitamin D absorption in laboratory rats. However, I soon became more interested in the fate of a very similar lipid (fatty substance), cholesterol, which was absorbed in an analogous manner to vitamin D and which was gaining prominence as a cause of atherosclerosis and coronary heart disease in man. This was in 1967, the year when Fredrickson and his colleagues at the National Institutes of Health (NIH) published a five-part monograph "Fat transport in Lipoproteins" in the *New England Journal of Medicine*.[5] This series of articles heralded the emergence of the embryonic specialty of lipidology as a clinical entity.

Also at the MGH was Neil McIntyre, and he, Hermon Dowling, the late Jim McManus, and I — a Welshman, an Irishman, a Scotsman, and an Englishman — were all research fellows in Boston at the same time and became firm friends. We all spoke the same language but I wasn't sure that all Americans did. It took me a while to interpret the meaning of "a submarine pastrami and a six pack to go." Americans in their turn were bemused when told that Hermon and I had imported Volvo saloons from Britain, saloons being synonymous with bars in the USA.

While I was at the MGH, I received a visit from Chris Booth who had just been appointed Professor of Medicine at the Hammersmith following the retirement of Sir John McMichael. Over lunch at the Union Oyster House he suggested I should apply for the vacant post of Lecturer in Gastroenterology, which carried Consultant status. The opportunity to become a member of staff at The Hammersmith was too good to miss so I applied and was duly appointed.

Boston to San Francisco and Back

The second half of the Sixties in the USA was dominated by the war in Vietnam, one consequence being the anti-war protests that were triggered by the introduction of the military draft in 1966. The succeeding years saw the heyday of the hippie movement with the "Summer of Love" in San Francisco and the LSD-fuelled Woodstock Festival. Martin Luther King and Robert Kennedy were both assassinated in 1968 but the decade ended on a more positive note with the landing of the first man on the moon, Neil Armstrong, by NASA's Apollo 11 in 1969.

Against this background and before we returned home to the UK, my wife and I and our two children set off in our Volvo, together with a tent and camping equipment, to drive from Boston to San Francisco and back, camping *en route*. It proved to be the hardest but best holiday of our lives and a marvellous way of seeing America. I did the driving and my wife did the cooking, with the aid of a Coleman stove. Our tent kept us dry apart from the time we camped in Muir Woods, near San Francisco, when the rain poured down all night long and we got soaked. This forced us to check into a motel the next day to dry out, much to our children's delight — it had a pool and TV in their bedroom.

We had started our trip by driving south from Boston to Philadelphia via New York, then going west on Interstate 70 to Colorado Springs. From there we veered southwest into Arizona, then northwest to San Francisco via the Grand Canyon, Las Vegas and Death Valley. The return trip took us eastwards to Salt Lake City, then north alongside the Grand Tetons, then east again into Yellowstone Park, where we camped. This was not entirely without risk because brown bears would sometimes forage for food in the tents.

While in Yellowstone I took the opportunity to fish the Firehole River, which is fed by hot springs and where, watched by bison in the woods behind me, I soon caught several rainbow trout (Figure 4). An American

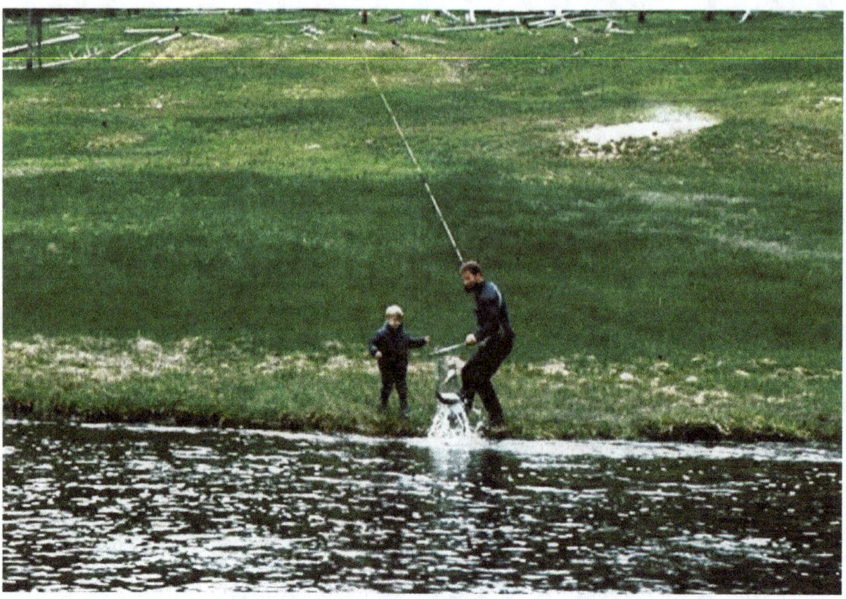

Figure 4. Success on the Firehole River, Yellowstone Park.

fisherman on the opposite bank was less successful, possibly because his casts landed like exploding depth charges. Eventually he called out to me "Say Bud, what 'yer catching 'em on?" I looked at my olive green fly and replied "A Large Olive." He looked perplexed for a moment and then said "D'yer reckon a small marshmallow might do?" Tongue in cheek I said I thought it might. Back in Britain many years later while having a drink at The Mayfly pub in Fullerton, I saw a large trout take a cocktail olive which had been thrown into the River Test by someone upstream — but I have yet to see one rise to a marshmallow.

Apart from a spectacular thunderstorm in the Badlands of South Dakota, the return journey was something of an anti-climax until we got to the Niagara Falls, which lived up to our expectations as had the Grand Canyon earlier on. From Niagara a final spurt through New York State brought us back to our house in Newton Upper Falls, just off Route 128, having covered almost 10,000 miles and acquired an unforgettable impression of the beauty and variety of the American landscape.

References

1. Thompson GR. A case of osteomalacia, osteoporosis and hypercalcaemia. *Br Med J* 1967;**i**:219–23.
2. Thompson GR, Lewis B, Booth CC. Absorption of vitamin D3-^{3}H in control subjects and patients with intestinal malabsorption. *J Clin Invest* 1966; **45**:94–102.
3. Thompson GR, Neale G, Watts JM, Booth CC. Detection of vitamin D deficiency after partial gastrectomy. *Lancet* 1966;**i**:623–6.
4. Thompson GR, Lewis B, Booth CC. Vitamin D absorption after partial gastrectomy. *Lancet* 1966;**i**:457–8.
5. Fredrickson DS, Levy RI, Lees RS. Fat transport in lipoproteins — an integrated approach to mechanisms and disorders. *N Engl J Med* 1967;34–44, 94–103, 148–56, 215–24, 273–81.

5 Texas

Post-Boston Blues

Re-entry to the Hammersmith environment after my time in Boston involved a long and difficult period of acclimatisation. I now had one of the most sought-after posts in gastroenterology in London but my heart was not in it. The specialty was becoming increasingly orientated towards endoscopy and the last thing I wanted was to spend the rest of my working life peering down into stomachs or up colons. Increasingly my interest was turning to lipids and atherosclerosis, which was not an appropriate line of research for a gastroenterologist. Nor was it easy "living in the shadow of the mountain" with Chris Booth in the Chair of Medicine at the Hammersmith further establishing his reputation as the leading academic in the specialty.

I compromised and undertook research into aspects of lipids which had gastroenterological connotations such as the lipid abnormalities found in patients with steatorrhoea, including essential fatty acid deficiency.[1] Diagnosis of the latter was by gas chromatography, which was performed by a Japanese research fellow who kept a bottle of Suntory whisky on the reagent shelf, to which he resorted when his gas chromatograph was misbehaving. However, the problem was that most gastrointestinal disorders lowered blood lipids whereas my real interest was in patients with raised levels. A research project that brought me closer to the latter objective was to investigate the mechanism whereby the antibiotic neomycin lowered serum cholesterol. This involved collaborating with Hermon Dowling to study its effect on fat absorption in humans[2] and, in conjunction with the Royal Veterinary College, in germ-free pigs.[3] Our results showed that neomycin impaired lipid absorption by disrupting micelle formation within the intestinal lumen via ionic interaction with fatty acids and bile acids, not because of its antibiotic properties.

While in Boston we had swapped houses with an American haematologist who had come to work at the Hammersmith. We kept in touch with each other after he went back to the States and in one of his letters he mentioned that Tony Gotto, who I'd met when he was an intern at the MGH, was moving from the NIH in Bethesda, where he'd been working with Don Fredrickson, to set up a lipoprotein research unit at the Methodist Hospital in Houston, Texas. I'd acquired a reasonable amount of expertise in lipid biochemistry but I lacked knowledge of the protein components of lipoproteins — termed apolipoproteins — a topic in which Tony excelled. Part of the funding of his new unit was from the Lipid Research Clinics (LRC) Program, an NIH venture aimed at determining the importance of hyperlipidaemia (raised blood lipid levels) as a cause of cardiovascular disease in the USA. The LRC Program was directed by Bob Levy, who was Don Fredrickson's right-hand man at the NIH. I'd met him in London previously and we soon became good friends. Tony persuaded him to provide a salary for me as an assistant professor at Baylor College of Medicine while I persuaded Chris Booth to grant me a year's leave of absence from the Hammersmith.

Houston

Hence in August 1972, my wife and I returned to the USA together with our 1-year-old son, leaving our two older children at boarding schools in England. Our destination, Houston, was considered the murder capital of the USA at that time and was the opposite in most respects to Boston. Houston was brash and modern but the local Texans were friendly with their inevitable "Y'all come back, now." It was more cosmopolitan than nearby Dallas, possibly reflecting the international nature of its main industry, oil. This was the year before OPEC disrupted the oil market and the city was booming, with new buildings springing up everywhere. Another boost to Houston's reputation came from the siting in nearby Pasadena of the Johnson Space Centre where Mission Control for the NASA space launches was located.

Despite the heat and humidity, reminiscent of Ghana, we soon settled in. All the houses had central air conditioning, as did most cars, so Houstonians seldom got too hot. I had imported a BMW without air conditioning so we did get hot whenever we went out for a drive. That is until I bought my wife a second-hand Buick Wildcat, a vast car with a leaky boot which accumulated so much rain water that it splashed like a swimming pool when in motion. But its air conditioning worked.

I enjoyed being back in the well-funded and rigorously scientific atmosphere that characterised American medical research and my project progressed well under Tony Gotto's supervision. At one stage this involved undertaking studies in volunteers from the local prison, which was permitted in the USA at that time. The two youths who volunteered to participate had been found guilty of taking peyote, a hallucinogenic cactus, and were serving a short jail sentence. They were remarkably cooperative and postponed their break for freedom until after the last blood sample had been taken. However, a policeman spotted them in the street in their pyjamas early the following morning, so they were soon back in prison.

Duck Shoot

As is well known, everything in Texas is on the tall side, including the people, their hats, and their stories. One of the fringe benefits of the Methodist Hospital was that it owned a large area of marsh near the coast and on one occasion a group of us arranged to go duck shooting there. We drove down to the edge of the marsh after work and then transferred to a speedboat, which delivered us to the shooting lodge's jetty where we were greeted with enormous Bloody Marys. After several of these the next item on the agenda was shooting practice at clays, a hilarious but hazardous activity. This was followed by a large dinner, rounded off with a game of poker which went on until well after midnight. No sooner had we got to bed, it seemed, than we were roused at 4 am to get ready for the duck shoot. We were conveyed to our hides in the marsh on airboats, metal punts each driven by an incredibly noisy aero-engine. This woke every duck in the place but since it was still pitch black, they stayed put. The hides were metal lined trenches, sunk into the marsh. The parting comments of my boatman were "Mind where you put yer feet, mister. Last guy I brought here trod on a water moccasin" and "Don't wander round lookin' for downed ducks or the alligators'll get you!"

Came the dawn and the ducks flew so the marsh soon sounded like a re-run of the battle of the Alamo. This lasted for an hour or so until the sun had risen and then the mosquitoes, looking almost as big as the ducks, began their attack. This meant it was time to contact the boatman by walkie-talkie, get back to the lodge for breakfast and return to Houston.

Galveston Beach and San Jacinto

A popular destination on weekends in the summer was the beach at Galveston on the Gulf of Mexico. The water looked like pea soup and was almost as warm. Our children loved it, the older two having flown over from England for their summer holidays. One drawback was that cars were allowed on the beach, which left patches of oil on the sand. Another was trying to stay awake on the six lane highway on the way home after a day in the sun, driving at a soporific 50 mph and listening to Country and Western music on the local radio station, much to my wife's disgust.

Another way of keeping the kids happy was to take them to visit the *USS Texas*, a decommissioned battleship berthed near the San Jacinto Monument, which soars skywards at the site of the battle it commemorates. This was where General Sam Houston defeated the Mexican General Santa Anna in 1836, thereby gaining Texas its independence and avenging the defeat at the Alamo. After exploring the ship with its huge 14-inch guns we gorged ourselves at a nearby restaurant, where for a few dollars each we could eat as many shrimps as we wanted (Figure 1). Oysters cost extra but that didn't deter an American colleague of mine who swallowed three dozen at one sitting without batting an eyelid.

Barbecues were a popular pastime in Texas and it was a custom we maintained after we returned to England. It so happened that my work in Houston necessitated raising antibodies to apoB, the protein component of low density lipoprotein (LDL). This involved repeatedly injecting de-lipidated LDL and a paraffin-based substance called Freund's adjuvant into two goats, with the objective of developing an immunoassay for quantifying apoB in human blood samples. Unfortunately, one of the goats ceased producing antibodies so we decided to cut our losses and despatch it humanely before barbecuing it on the beach at Galveston, using the discarded bonnet of a Volkswagen Beetle as a make-shift baking tray. The haunch I ate must have

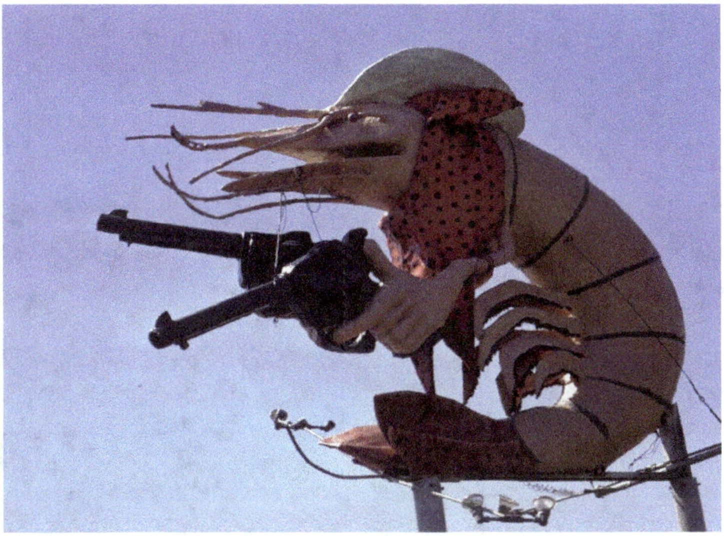

Figure 1. Sign outside a seafood restaurant, Houston.

been the site of injection of the Freund's adjuvant because it tasted revolting. Later we had the goat's horned head stuffed and mounted on a plaque inscribed "Goatto" and we presented it to Tony Gotto, who accepted it with his usual sangfroid. He had been a Rhodes Scholar at Oxford so knew that the British had an odd sense of humour.

Houston was not just a city of high-rise, glass-fronted buildings although it had plenty of these. Some of the residential roads had evocative names such as Old Spanish Trail and Buffalo Speedway and were lined with low profile, spacious houses. Rivers were called bayous (Figure 2) and their banks were pleasant places to jog, a habit I first acquired there. I used to do this in the cool of the evenings and not, like an elderly Houstonian pouring sweat, in the midday sun. I later discovered that his personalised number plate was "I RUN 11" which apparently referred to his daily mileage.

A Camping Trip Around Texas

In April 1973, my wife and I and our 3 children decided to spend 10 days camping our way around Texas, much as we had done on our trip across

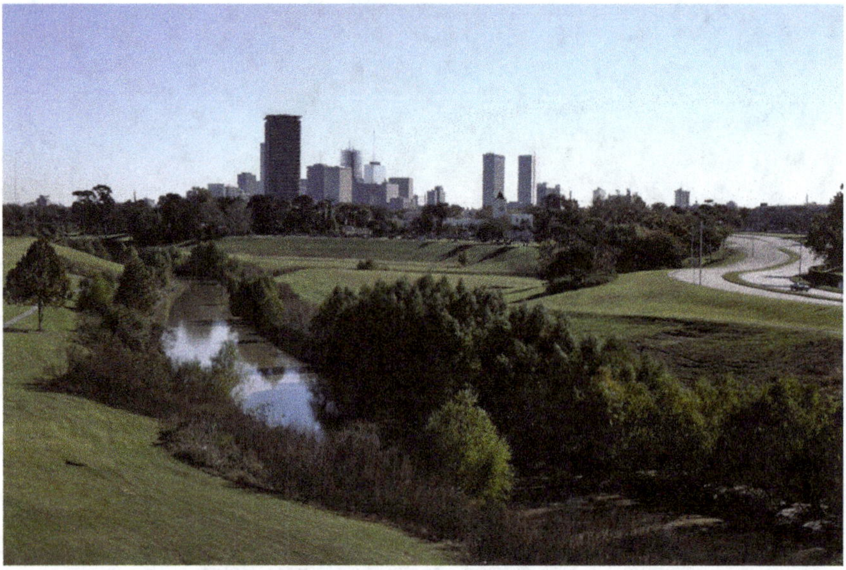

Figure 2. Downtown Houston seen from Buffalo Bayou in 1973.

the USA 6 years previously. We started off from Houston in our BMW and drove north via Austin, the state capital, then through Archer City, the town that featured in the film of the book *The Last Picture Show*. By-passing Wichita Falls we then headed west and drove across the high plains of the Texas Panhandle to Amarillo, where we camped in Palo Duro Canyon. We had the entire place to ourselves apart from the racoons, which kept us awake with the noise they made raiding the camp site's dustbins. The canyon's most striking feature is a sandstone pinnacle called the Lighthouse, to the base of which the two older children climbed. Amarillo is located in the north-west corner of Texas, sandwiched between Oklahoma to the east and New Mexico to the west, and it used to be a major cattle marketing centre. From there we drove south down a seemingly endless, straight and empty highway to the Monahans, an area of sand dunes in West Texas where we camped and where our youngest revelled in the soft sand. We then headed for Big Bend National Park, passing the formidable El Capitan (8085 ft), which stands in the Guadalupe Mountains National Park and is not to be confused with its more famous namesake in Yosemite National Park in California. Once we reached Big Bend we waded across

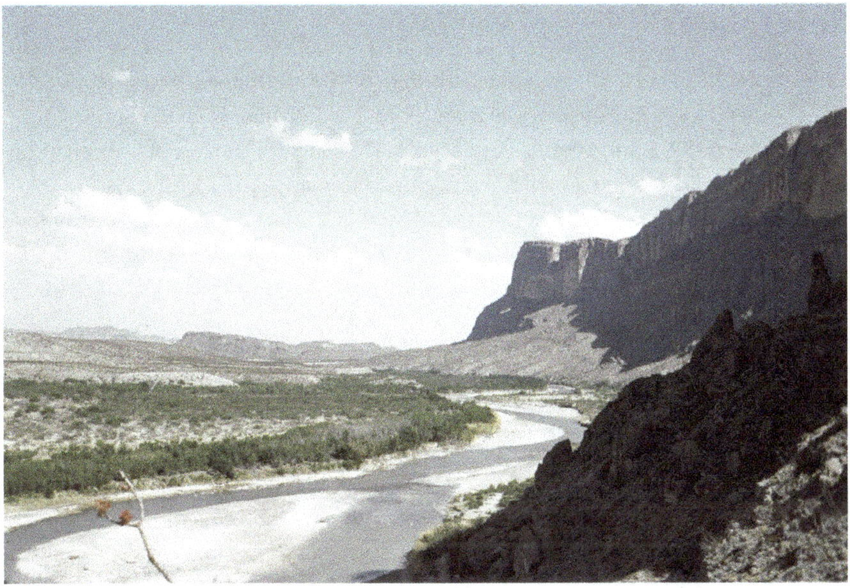

Figure 3. The Rio Grande with Mexico on the right bank and Texas on the left.

the Rio Grande (Figure 3) and up into the Santa Elena canyon, in all probability making an illegal crossing into Mexico! The giant yuccas in the desert were in full bloom and were very spectacular. After camping in Big Bend we then went eastwards, stopping off to visit the movie set at Bracketville, where the film *The Alamo* was shot as well as numerous other Westerns. We then drove back to Houston via San Antonio, where we stopped off to visit the ruins of the real Alamo, where Travis, Crockett, and Bowie reputedly fought to the death in the face of overwhelming odds and became legendary Texan heroes.

I managed to get my leave of absence extended for 3 months after we got back from our trip but all too soon it was time to return to London. Our arrival home at the end of 1973 coincided with the OPEC oil crisis, when cars queued up outside petrol stations and life in Britain was at its most difficult, an ominous portent for the next stage of my career. Nevertheless my time in Houston had not been wasted; I had made many good friends during my stay there and acquired valuable knowledge and skills. The question was, would I have the opportunity to use the latter to good effect after my return home?

References

1. Press M, Kikuchi H, Shimoyama T, Thompson GR. Diagnosis and treatment of essential fatty acid deficiency in man. *Br Med J* 1974;**ii**:247–50.
2. Thompson GR, Barrowman J, Gutierrez L, Dowling RH. Action of neomycin on the intraluminal phase of lipid absorption. *J Clin Invest* 1971;**50**:319–23.
3. Thompson GR, Henry K, Edington N, Trexler PC. Effect of neomycin on cholesterol metabolism in the germ-free pig. *Eur J Clin Invest* 1972;**2**:365–71.

6 "A Bloody Great Swerve" in Mid-Career

In Limbo

"Nature abhors a vacuum" proved an appropriate adage for my return to the Hammersmith because all the office and laboratory space in the gastroenterology unit was occupied. Instead, it was arranged that I should be accommodated in the cardiovascular research unit, where Professor Jack Shillingford kindly provided me with some temporary office space. While there I spent my time catching up with the burgeoning literature on lipids and lipoproteins and building up a card index of references. Chris Booth was probably hoping that Jack might be willing to take me off his hands but this proved illusory. The latter's concept of cardiovascular research did not include lipids: "A low fat diet won't make you live longer, it will just make life seem longer" was one of his favourite aphorisms.

My main objective at this stage was to quit gastroenterology and move into the lipid field, so as to resume the type of work I'd been doing in Houston. However, my discussions with Chris Booth reached an impasse and it seemed that the only way of achieving my objective would be to emigrate. I entered into discussions with Tony Gotto about getting a permanent position in Houston. The prospects looked encouraging and 6 months after my return to London I sent in my letter of resignation to the dean of the Royal Postgraduate Medical School. In retrospect, this was distinctly foolhardy because I did not have any definite prospect of an alternative source of income. Fortunately, Chris Booth kindly kept me on the payroll to give me time to sort out my future.

Yudkin's Sugar Hypothesis

This all took place in June 1974, at a time when my chances of continuing to work in Britain appeared bleak. However, "it's always darkest before the dawn" and the very next month an article appeared in *The Times* with the title "Why suspicion falls on sugar as a major cause of heart disease."[1] The author was John Yudkin, Emeritus Professor of Nutrition at King's College, London and in the article he challenged orthodox views on the role of diet in the causation of coronary heart disease.

The article was provocative in that it criticised the basic tenets of the lipid hypothesis of atherosclerosis by suggesting that excess dietary sugar, which raised serum triglycerides, was more important than an increased intake of saturated fat in the diet, which raised serum cholesterol, in causing atherosclerosis and coronary heart disease. Yudkin began his article by pointing out that not a single statement could be made about coronary heart disease that would not be contradicted by someone. Taking him at his word I persuaded *The Times* to publish my rebuttal of his views, under the title "Beware sweet reason in the search for causes of heart disease."[2] In my article, I quoted Martin Fischer: "Don't confuse hypothesis and theory. The former is a possible explanation; the latter the correct one." I went on to assert that the evidence supporting the saturated fat theory was causal whereas that supporting the sugar hypothesis was circumstantial.

Yudkin had previously reported that the increase in coronary disease in Britain was proportional to the increase in radio and television licences and he suggested that the evidence linking saturated fat, serum cholesterol, and coronary disease was in a similar category, lacking proof of causality. In particular, the lack of evidence from dietary trials that modifying fat intake reduces the risk of coronary heart disease made him conclude that the lipid hypothesis was defunct. Among the alternative explanations he proposed were an excess of protein, carbohydrate, or sugar in the diet.[3]

Consumption of sugar in Britain had increased 25-fold during the past 200 years, and Yudkin cited data that a high intake of sucrose could raise serum cholesterol and triglyceride, especially the latter, as well as levels of insulin, cortisol, and uric acid, and that it also impaired glucose tolerance and induced a clotting tendency. He claimed that all these abnormalities were evident in subjects with coronary disease and he proposed that they reflected a hormonal disturbance brought about by excessive consumption of sucrose. He concluded that eating less sugar would correct the hormonal imbalance and also favourably influence dental disease, diabetes, and obesity, whereas altering dietary fat intake, particularly increasing the intake of polyunsaturated fats, would achieve none of these objectives and might have adverse side effects.

Earlier in 1974, Yudkin had contributed to a Report of the Committee on Medical Aspects (COMA) of Food Policy on diet in relation to cardiovascular disease.[4] The majority of the other members of the committee recommended that the amount of total and saturated fat in the UK diet should be reduced to decrease cardiovascular disease and that sucrose consumption should be reduced to decrease obesity. However, in a note of reservation at the end of the report, Yudkin recorded his opinion that the role of dietary fat in causing cardiovascular disease had been exaggerated and that the role of sucrose had been minimized. One of the other members of the committee, JRA Mitchell, was subsequently highly critical of Yudkin, especially his citing as evidence theoretical speculations bearing no proven relationship to the matter under discussion.[5]

Yudkin's claims regarding the link between sugar and vascular disease were based on remarkably scanty experimental evidence. In 1964, he and Roddy had shown that the estimated intake of sucrose in 45 men with coronary or peripheral vascular disease was significantly greater than that of 25 controls.[6] On the basis of these results they claimed that the relationship between sucrose and vascular disease was causal and that people taking over 110 g/day were five times more likely to develop myocardial infarction than those taking under 60 g/day. Three years later, following criticisms of the methodology used to estimate sucrose intake, Yudkin and Morland carried out another study, modified so as to minimize any bias in estimating dietary intake, in 20 myocardial infarct survivors and 33 controls, and again found a significantly higher intake of sucrose among the former.[7]

In the light of these findings, the MRC convened a working party to investigate the relationship between sugar and vascular disease. Studies were performed in four centres, two in London and two in Scotland. The largest study took place at the Central Middlesex Hospital in London and another was conducted at the Edinburgh Royal Infirmary. The pooled results of all these studies showed no difference between the sucrose intake of 122 myocardial infarct survivors and 113 controls, leading the working party to conclude, in 1970, "The evidence in favour of a high sugar intake as a major factor in the development of myocardial infarction is extremely slender."[8]

BBC TV Debate

This conflict of views came to the attention of the producer of the BBC series "Controversy" who invited Don Fredrickson, assisted by the Middlesex Hospital cardiologist Peter Taggart and myself, to participate in a televised debate with John Yudkin on the topic "The dietary cause of heart disease is sugar not fat." Fredrickson agreed to fly over from the USA and the event duly took place in early September 1974 at the Royal Institution and was chaired by the Nobel Laureate Sir George Porter.

Despite being outnumbered 3 to 1, Yudkin put up a stiff resistance and kept bouncing back like a punch ball after repeated verbal knockdowns (Figure 1). Although he was wrong in suggesting that sugar not fat was a direct cause of heart disease, he was correct in pointing out the danger of excessive

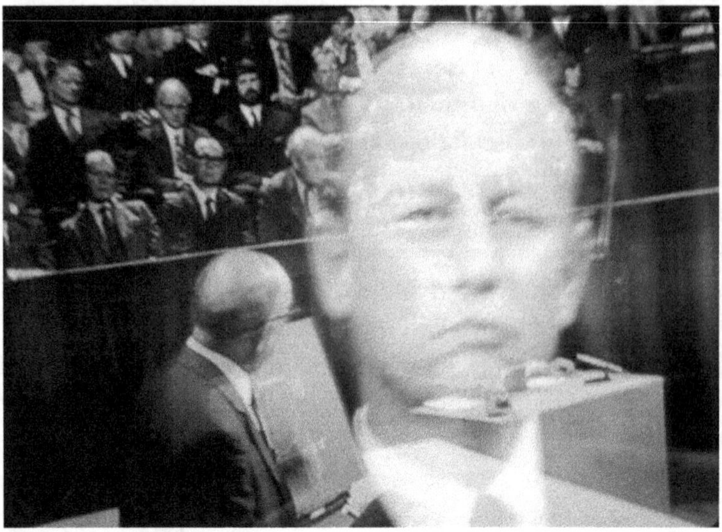

Figure 1. Double take of TV debate between Don Fredrickson (1924–2002) (right) and John Yudkin (1910–1995) (left).

sugar intake as an indirect cause by inducing obesity and type 2 diabetes, both of which predispose affected individuals to develop coronary heart disease. Following the debate, Don Fredrickson and I had dinner together in a nearby restaurant. At that stage he was president of the Institute of Medicine of the National Academy of Sciences in Washington and about to become director of the NIH, although one would never have guessed it from his unassuming manner. In the latter role, he soon became involved in another controversy, over recombinant DNA research, and was instrumental in getting this legitimized in the face of considerable opposition. He was a man of great charm and wit, the exception that proves the rule that "nice guys finish last!"

In retrospect, the biochemical abnormalities which Yudkin attributed to excess sugar consumption have now become recognized as being part of the metabolic syndrome. The latter is an accompaniment of the central obesity which is becoming increasingly common nowadays as a result of excessive caloric intake, especially when derived from rapidly absorbed carbohydrate. Individuals with the metabolic syndrome have an increased liability to develop coronary heart disease, so in this respect Yudkin was right. Where he erred was in overemphasizing the role of sucrose, despite the evidence against it, and in disregarding the role of saturated fat, despite the evidence for it. Official acceptance of his views on dietary fat could have had unforeseen consequences for the population approach to prevention of coronary heart disease in Britain, but, happily, this was avoided. The only reference to sugar in the subsequent recommendations from COMA 10 years later regarding cardiovascular prevention was that the intake of sucrose, glucose, and fructose should not increase any further.[9]

Yudkin's views on diet and heart disease must have been music to the ears of the National Dairy Council. The late Keith Ball, one of the earliest advocates of dietary change to prevent coronary disease, criticized the massive advertising campaign conducted by the Butter Information Council and the National Dairy Council to persuade doctors and the public to disregard official advice to reduce saturated fat intake.[10] He claimed that general practitioners had been circulated with the names of experts who disagreed with the views expressed by official bodies such as COMA, and he questioned the ethics of such promotional activities. Yudkin himself, of course, had openly dissociated himself from COMA's views on fat intake while he was a member of the committee in 1974.

John Yudkin died in 1995 and will be remembered not just for his views on sucrose but also as the holder of the first Chair of Nutrition in the UK, established at Queen Elizabeth College, which later honoured him by making him a Fellow. He was highly regarded in nutrition circles and were he alive today he would have been pleased that the latest American College of Cardiology/American Heart Association guideline on the primary prevention of cardiovascular disease recommends minimising the dietary intake of refined carbohydrates and sweetened beverages.[11]

The BBC debate sparked considerable interest and strengthened my resolve to study the role of lipids in atherosclerosis, preferably in Britain where there was a dearth of research on this topic compared with the USA. I received considerable encouragement in this ambition from Nick Myant, Director of the MRC Lipid Metabolism Unit at the Hammersmith. I had first come into contact with him 10 years previously via a member of his unit, Barry Lewis, with whom I had collaborated in developing the vitamin D absorption test. He and Nick had set up the first lipid clinic in Britain at the Hammersmith and I used to assist them in seeing patients with lipid abnormalities both before and after my time in Houston. Nick had a special interest in familial hypercholesterolaemia (FH) and we followed up the patients with this disorder who were referred to him at the lipid clinic. These included two young women with extremely high cholesterol levels and coronary heart disease due to homozygous FH (i.e. each had inherited two mutant alleles, one from each parent), a very rare and usually fatal condition that was refractory to all forms of cholesterol-lowering therapy available at the time.

First Use of Plasma Exchange in Homozygous FH

In collaboration with an Australian haematology registrar, Ray Lowenthal, Nick Myant and I decided to treat the two FH homozygotes with plasma exchange, a novel and radical approach that involved removing their hyper-cholesterolaemic plasma from a vein in one arm and replacing it with an equal volume of a cholesterol-free albumin solution via a vein in the other arm, using a device known as a continuous flow centrifugal cell separator to separate the plasma from blood cells, discard the plasma, and then return the blood cells and albumin to the patient (Figure 2). Despite our anxieties

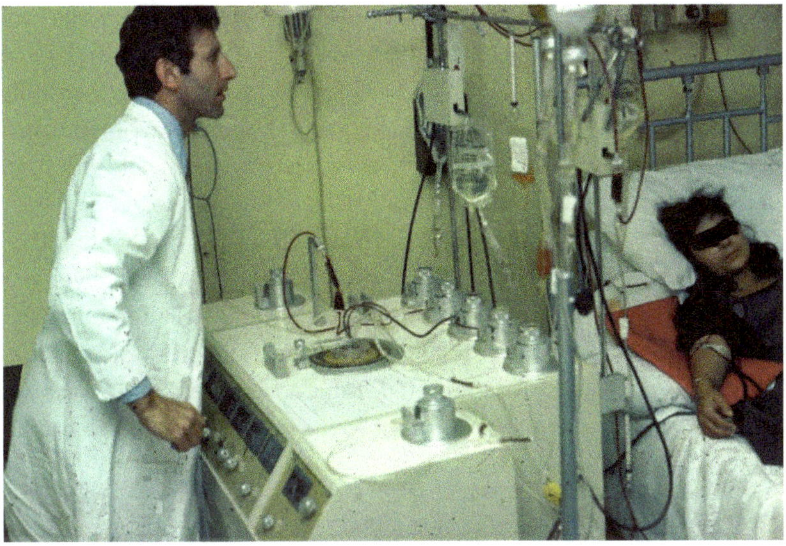

Figure 2. First patient with homozygous familial hypercholesterolaemia undergoing plasma exchange in 1974.

that it might precipitate their angina both patients tolerated this procedure (during which they were anti-coagulated with heparin) remarkably well and it resulted in unprecedentedly large reductions in their cholesterol levels. We therefore continued to plasma exchange them at 2 weekly intervals for 6 months and then published our findings in *The Lancet* in 1975.[12] The article had an immediate impact and plasma exchange was soon adopted by other centres including the NIH. It also led to several reports in newspapers and magazines here and abroad including one in *New Scientist* titled "Swopping plasma to reduce cholesterol" and to my appearing on the BBC programme *Tomorrow's World*. Tragically, the first of the two patients we had treated died a short while later during a coronary artery bypass operation, aged 23, but the other lived into her 50s. Now, more than 40 years later, an improved version of plasma exchange known as lipoprotein apheresis remains an effective and safe first line treatment for homozygous FH.

Presenting such patients on the Staff Round provided useful publicity and the Royal Postgraduate Medical School re-instated my senior lectureship until I could find an alternative source of funding. Nick Myant was very supportive and persuaded the MRC to let me join his Unit as a member of the external scientific staff, starting in May 1975. The preceding year had proved to be a watershed in my career and henceforth my energies were devoted solely to clinical research into lipids. This increasingly brought me into contact, and occasionally conflict, with cardiologists, whose patients often manifested the cardiovascular complications of untreated hyperlipidaemia. Chief among those who were supportive was the Hammersmith cardiologist Celia Oakley, a feisty red head, who provided the expertise needed for the management of the complex cardiac problems posed by patients with FH, especially those with the homozygous form of the disorder. However, much of the cardiology establishment remained apathetic or in some instances positively antagonistic to the concept that lipids played a role in atherosclerosis. The persistence of the latter attitude in at least one cardiologist was exemplified by a referral letter sent to me by a GP a dozen years later:

> Mr S is a 38 year old man who underwent an extensive coronary artery bypass operation in December 1987. His post-operative recovery was physically uneventful. However, we were quite concerned about our inability to reduce his high cholesterol and triglyceride levels. Up until August 1988 he was taking Questran (cholestyramine) six a day and Maxepa (fish oil) 5 mL bd (twice daily). On that regime, his cholesterols were 8.4–9.5 mmol/L and triglycerides 3.3–5.3 mmol/L. Mr S was getting very 'screwed up' about his inability to drop his cholesterol and triglycerides and was very frightened that his new coronary arteries were soon to get furred up. As a result of this, I referred him to the Brompton Hospital. He saw a consultant who told him to forget taking any tablets, to forget his cholesterol and triglycerides and to go away and try and live a normal life. That advice caused us some considerable concern, especially as we have been working very hard on him over the past couple of years to reduce these levels. He is now on no medication.

The Brompton was and still is regarded as the premier cardiac centre in London so hopefully the negative attitude of the consultant concerned was the exception and not the rule.

Workshop on FH

Reverting back to 1975, in view of his long-standing interest in FH and because of recent progress in knowledge of the cause and treatment of the disease, Nick and I decided to organise a meeting on the topic. This took

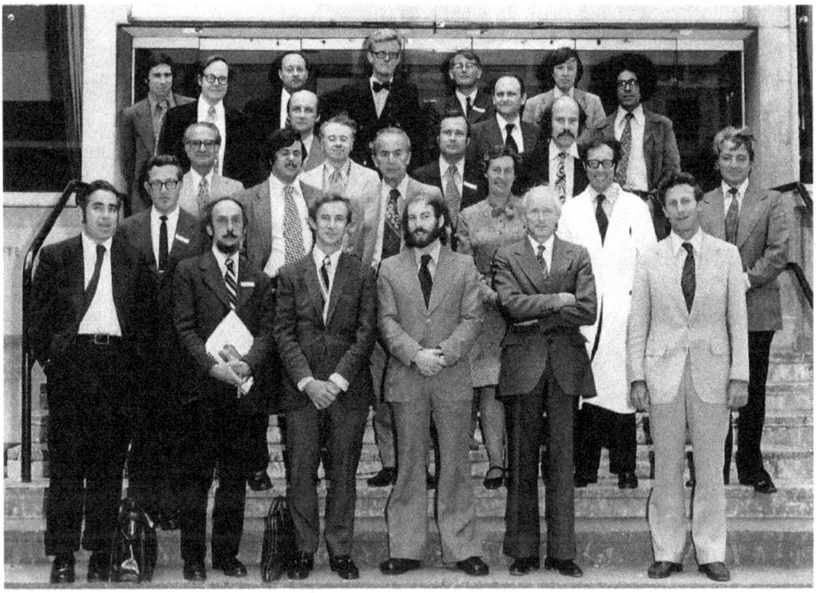

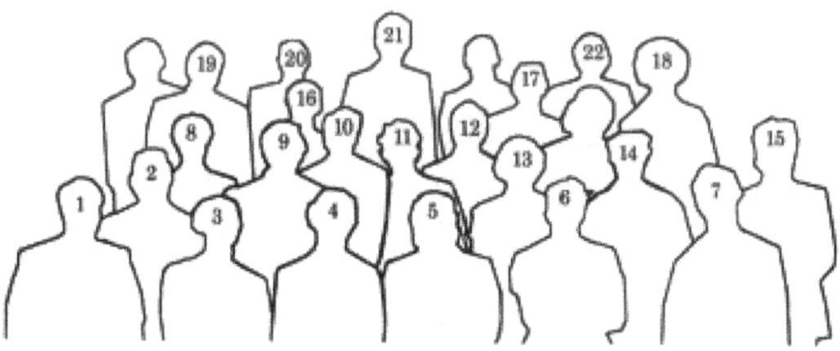

Key:

1 = R. Levy; 2 = R. Lees; 3 = D. Steinberg; 4 = A. Gotto; 5 = M. Press; 6 = N. Myant; 7 = G. Thompson; 8 = A. Khachadurian; 9 = M. Brown; 10 = J. Goldstein; 11 = G. Popjak; 12 = D. Bilheimer; 13 = J. Slack; 14 = B. Lewis; 15 = K. Mitropoulos; 16 = T. Miettinen; 17 = D. Reichl; 18 = H. Magnani; 19 = S. Grundy; 20 = J. de Gennes; 21 = K. Hellstrom; 22 = G. Gibbons.

Figure 3. Participants in meeting on FH at Hammersmith Hospital in 1975.

place at the Hammersmith in September that year and we invited most of the leading figures in lipid research in the USA and Europe (Figure 3). Nearly all of them agreed to attend apart from Don Fredrickson, who had other commitments. They included Joe Goldstein, Mike Brown, Tony Gotto, Dan Steinberg, Bob Levy, George Popjak, Scott Grundy, and many others, all of them household names in the world of lipid research. The meeting was just the right size and at the right time and proved to be an outstanding success. It helped re-inforce my belief that I was on the right track and that at last I was starting to make some progress. In the words of Robert Frost "I took the road less travelled by and that made all the difference."

References

1. Yudkin J. Why suspicion falls on sugar as a major cause of heart disease. *The Times* 1974; 11 July, p. 16.
2. Thompson GR. Beware sweet reason in the search for causes of heart disease. *The Times* 1974; 31 July, p.16.
3. Yudkin J. Sucrose and cardiovascular disease. *Proc Nutr Soc* 1972;**31**:331–7.
4. Department of Health and Social Security. Diet and coronary heart disease: Report of the Advisory Panel of the Committee on Medical Aspects of Food Policy (Nutrition) on diet in relation to cardiovascular and cerebrovascular disease. London: HMSO 1974 (Report on Health and Social Subjects, no. 7).
5. Mitchell JRA. Diet and coronary heart disease — a British point of view. *Adv Exp Med Biol* 1977;**82**:823–7.
6. Yudkin J, Roddy J. Levels of dietary sucrose in patients with occlusive atherosclerotic disease. *Lancet* 1964;**41**:6–8.
7. Yudkin J, Morland J. Sugar intake and myocardial infarction. *Am J Clin Nutr* 1967;**20**:503–6.
8. Dietary sugar intake in men with myocardial infarction. Report to the Medical Research Council by its working party on the relationship between dietary sugar intake and arterial disease. *Lancet* 1970;**2**:1265–71.
9. Department of Health and Social Security. Diet and Cardiovascular Disease: Report of the Panel on Diet in Relation to Cardiovascular Disease, Committee on Medical Aspects of Food Policy. London: HMSO, 1984 (Report on Health and Social Subjects, no. 28).
10. Ball K. Prevention of coronary heart-disease. *Lancet* 1979;**2**:1182.
11. Arnett DK, Blumenthal RS, Albert MA *et al*. 2019 ACC/AHA Guideline on the Primary Prevention of Cardiovascular Disease: Executive Summary: A Report of the American College of Cardiology/American Heart Association Task Force on Clinical Practice Guidelines. *J Am Coll Cardiol*. 2019;74:e177–e232. doi: 10.1016/j.jacc.2019.03.009.
12. Thompson GR, Lowenthal R, Myant NB. Plasma exchange in the management of homozygous familial hypercholesterolaemia. *Lancet* 1975;**i**:1208–11.

7 The Origins of Clinical Lipidology

The Controversy Over Cholesterol

It is hard to be definite about the source of the cholesterol controversy in Britain, but it might have been the competitive environment that existed in the Postgraduate Medical School at Hammersmith Hospital after the Second World War. The Department of Medicine there was dominated by cardiologists, the most notable being John McMichael, the Professor of Medicine, and his first assistants Paul Wood and Peter Sharpey-Schafer. Legendary altercations reputedly took place between Sharpey-Schafer, educated at Winchester, King's College, Cambridge, and University College Hospital, London, and Wood, who had trained in Melbourne and had an Antipodean lack of respect for the Establishment.[1] Like his famous grandfather, Sir Edward Sharpey-Schafer FRS, Sharpey-Schafer was intolerant of those he considered intellectually inferior,[2] whereas Wood was scornful of his colleague's lack of clinical experience in cardiology.

Sharpey-Schafer left the Hammersmith scene in 1948 when he was appointed Professor of Medicine at St. Thomas's Hospital. As a medical student there I remember attending a ward round that he conducted in complete silence, his sole interest seemingly being to inspect his patients' necks to ascertain which of them had a raised jugular venous pressure (a sign of heart failure). His death in 1963, aged only 55, was described by McMichael as a unique loss.[2]

Paul Wood left the Hammersmith a year after Sharpey-Schafer, in 1949, when he was invited to set up the Institute of Cardiology at the National Heart Hospital and teach clinical cardiology to postgraduates.

His book *Diseases of the Heart and Circulation*, published in 1950, was mandatory reading for anyone aspiring to pass the MRCP exam. According to Michael Oliver,[3] the first edition contained the earliest British reference to the relationship between cholesterol and coronary heart disease, namely that "considerations should be given to the possibility that raised cholesterol might result from coronary heart disease." This comment probably reflected Wood's preoccupation with the manifestations of cardiac disease rather than its causes.

Lipids "Irrelevant to Cardiology"

In 1953, Michael Oliver, then a young cardiologist at the Edinburgh Royal Infirmary, and George Boyd, a biochemist at Edinburgh University, reported the findings of a study of 200 patients with coronary disease and an equal number of control subjects at a meeting of the British Cardiac Society in Newcastle. Their results showed that plasma cholesterol levels were significantly higher in the coronary patients, the first time this had been demonstrated in the UK. However, there was total silence after Oliver's presentation, and not a single question was asked during the discussion period. The silence was broken eventually by Paul Wood, who commented that this was irrelevant to cardiology.[4] That remark reflected the abrasively intolerant side of Wood's character, although he had many compensatory virtues,[1] while the absence of questions from the audience illustrated the complete lack of interest in lipids among British cardiologists at that time.

Undeterred, Oliver and Boyd pursued their research into lipids, using paper electrophoresis to separate the different classes of lipoproteins present in serum. They showed that patients with coronary disease not only had higher levels of total cholesterol than controls[5] but also that its distribution within the lipoprotein classes was abnormal, with an excess of β-lipoprotein and a dearth of α-lipoprotein.[6] In today's jargon, their patients had a raised level of low density lipoprotein (LDL) and a decreased level of high density lipoprotein (HDL). Both are now well accepted as risk factors for coronary disease, positive and negative, respectively, but these were novel findings at the time. However, their next research venture was less successful, involving the administration of oestrogens to men with coronary disease. Although this treatment lowered serum cholesterol, it had feminizing side effects and failed to reduce coronary events.[7]

Paul Wood and George Boyd both died from coronary disease before they reached 60, an all too common event in those days. Wood had explicitly stated that he was not to be resuscitated, and therefore no attempt to do so was made when he had a cardiac arrest. The photograph of him in the published account of the first Paul Wood Lecture, established in his honour by the British Cardiac Society (now British Cardiovascular Society), shows a lean, quizzical-looking man holding a tell-tale cigarette between his fingers.[1] His death in 1962 at the age of 55 shocked cardiologists across the country, but, as he himself had said, he enjoyed living dangerously. He took risks and unfortunately paid the price.

Edinburgh was not the only centre where lipid-orientated research in Britain was undertaken during the 1950s, another being Oxford. Brian Bronte-Stewart, a Cape Town graduate, was one of several immigrants from South Africa who made contributions to atherosclerosis research in Britain. When he first arrived, he worked with George Pickering at St. Mary's Hospital in London, but moved to Oxford in 1956 with Pickering when the latter was appointed Regius Professor. Bronte-Stewart's previous research was in Cape Town, where he and Ancel Keys demonstrated differences in serum cholesterol between racial groups, which they attributed to differences in animal fat intake. Bronte-Stewart went on to show that differing death rates from coronary heart disease in various European countries, including Britain, correlated better with the solid:liquid fat ratio of the diet than with the total fat intake.[8] He also showed that when vegetable oils are hydrogenated (hardened) they lose their cholesterol-lowering ability. In 1961, he was appointed director of the newly established MRC Atheroma Research Unit in Glasgow, but he tragically died from cancer 4 years later, aged only 42.

Another researcher in Oxford was Hugh Sinclair, an engagingly eccentric Fellow of Magdalen College, who was Reader in Human Nutrition and directed the Laboratory of Human Nutrition there for many years. In 1972, he established the International Institute of Human Nutrition on his estate at Sutton Courtenay, Abingdon. He, too, was interested in the role of diet in atherosclerosis but did not subscribe to the orthodox dogma that a high-fat diet caused a high serum cholesterol. His conflicting views on this issue are discussed in Chapter 10.

Role of Epidemiology Rejected

Apart from lipidology, another discipline that got short shrift from the Hammersmith cardiologists was epidemiology. The two may in fact have been unpopular for the same reason, in that both involved measurements performed in large groups or populations rather than individuals. This was the dawn of cardiac catheterization, and McMichael and his colleagues boldly exploited the technique to advance knowledge of cardiovascular haemodynamics by undertaking detailed studies in small numbers of subjects. To their minds, that was how real clinical research should be conducted. In contrast, Maurice Pappworth considered that some of the clinical research conducted at the Hammersmith during that era was unethical and detailed his criticisms in his book *Human Guinea Pigs.*[9]

In 1953, Jerry Morris, then director of the MRC Social Medicine Unit and regarded by many as the founding father of cardiovascular epidemiology in Britain, came up with some novel findings which suggested a link between coronary disease and exercise at work. He and his colleagues discovered that fatal heart attacks occurred less frequently in London bus conductors than in drivers and less often in postmen than in sedentary civil servants, findings which created a considerable stir when they were published.[10,11] Before they came out, however, he was advised by the secretary of the MRC, Sir Harold Himsworth, to show the data to John McMichael. He did so and went on to suggest that epidemiology could play a useful role in supplementing clinical observation and laboratory experiments. According to Morris, McMichael listened carefully until he had finished and then retorted "Rubbish!"[12] In sharp contrast, the director of the US National Heart and Lung Institute flew over from Bethesda, Maryland, to discuss the possibility of a follow-up study, and Paul Dudley White, the doyen of American cardiologists, phoned from Boston to congratulate him. Morris stated that McMichael "came round in later years,"[11] but there was no sign of this 20 years later, when he again rejected the concept that exercise had a protective effect and criticized "the unfortunate separation of epidemiology from close clinical analysis of the data," the implication being that only the latter could reveal causal relationships.

This, then, was the uncompromising environment confronting those interested in carrying out research into atherosclerosis and coronary disease in Britain at the start of the 1960s. Although the statistics showed that this disorder was the commonest cause of death in both men and women, little was done in the way of prevention apart from discouraging smoking. The only other risk factor taken seriously was blood pressure, hypertension being a topic of particular interest to McMichael at the Hammersmith and to Pickering at Oxford. The 1950s and 1960s were the heyday of clinicians in the National Health Service, who effectively ran it, and at the top of the tree were academic cardiologists such as McMichael and Pickering.

Early Research into Lipids in the UK

Unlike most clinicians, basic scientists in 20th century Britain took seriously research into lipids in general and cholesterol in particular. In contrast, lipidology was regarded as a minor branch of chemical pathology, and not a subject with which any practising clinician would wish to become involved. It remains a subspecialty, but nowadays the importance of a working knowledge of lipids in the management and prevention of cardiovascular disease is widely acknowledged.

Alistair Frazer, Head of the Department of Medical Biochemistry and Pharmacology at the University of Birmingham in the 1950s, arguably can be regarded as the founding father of clinical lipidology in Britain. His main interests were the mechanism of lipid absorption and the malabsorption of dietary fat associated with intestinal disorders such as tropical sprue, coeliac disease, and idiopathic steatorrhoea. He was a large man, and this together with his scientific interests led to his being known as "Fats" Frazer. In his introduction to an issue of the *British Medical Bulletin* in 1958 devoted to the metabolism of lipids, Frazer stated, "Agreement has not been reached on the precise aetiological relationship between blood lipids and atheroma, although few would deny its existence."[13] As it transpired, he was right on the first count, but not on the second.

One of the more notable contributions to that issue of the *British Medical Bulletin* was a paper on the biosynthesis of cholesterol by Cornforth and Popjak; the former was later to receive the Nobel Prize in Chemistry and a knighthood for his research on that topic. His co-author, George Popjak, was Head of the MRC Experimental Radiopathology Unit at Hammersmith Hospital at the time, and some thought he should have shared the Nobel Prize with Cornforth. In 1953, Popjak's unit was joined by Nick Myant, who had been a house physician to both Sir Thomas Lewis (during the war) and John McMichael (after the war). Subsequently, he embarked on a lifelong career with the MRC, first at University College Hospital and then at the Hammersmith. Myant recalled that Popjak was convinced of the validity of the lipid hypothesis and considered that understanding cholesterol synthesis would contribute to the treatment of coronary heart disease[14]: how right this later proved to be.

When Popjak left the Hammersmith in 1962, Myant joined the external staff of the MRC. At that stage, his main research interest was the thyroid gland, including the effect of thyroxine on cholesterol synthesis and the treatment of thyrotoxicosis (over activity of the thyroid gland) with radioactive iodine (^{131}I). In 1963, he was joined by Barry Lewis from Cape Town, a contemporary of Bronte-Stewart, who had previously undertaken research on lipids in South Africa and then at St. George's Hospital in London. After Lewis's arrival at Hammersmith, Myant's research activities became more lipid oriented and clinical, the latter facilitated by his being given access to four beds within the hospital. Together they set up an outpatient lipid clinic, the first in Britain, and began to undertake research into the regulation of cholesterol metabolism and the treatment of patients with FH.

Myant remained a member of the external staff of the MRC at Hammersmith until 1969, when space became available in the Cyclotron Unit. His group was then reconstituted as the MRC Lipid Metabolism Unit, which I joined in 1975, and which he directed until he retired in 1983. During that period, the main focus of his research was FH, the association of which with coronary disease had been first described by the Norwegian physician, Müller.[15] This disorder exemplifies Robert Frost's comment, "Nature is always hinting at us," namely that the presence of hypercholesterolaemia from birth onwards results in premature atherosclerosis and cardiovascular disease. Myant was especially interested in the mechanism of the hypercholesterolaemia in FH, and he undertook studies of the turnover of ^{14}C-labelled cholesterol to determine whether increased synthesis or decreased catabolism of cholesterol was responsible, but with inconclusive results.[16]

During the ensuing years, Nick Myant had a major influence on lipid research in Britain and was regarded with affectionate respect by all who

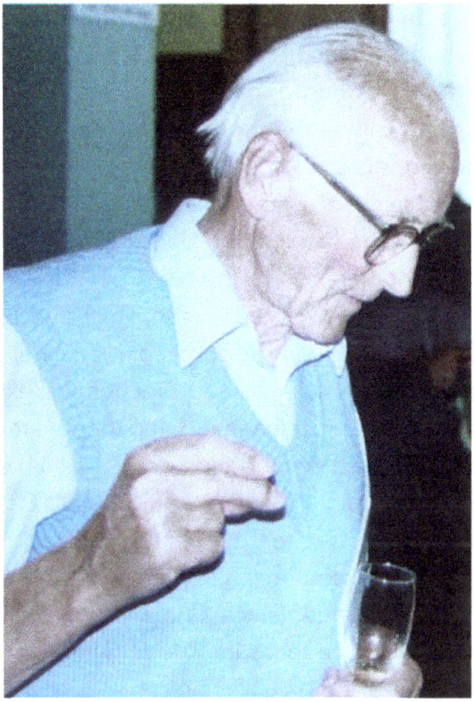

Figure 1. Nick Myant (1917–2015).

worked with him, and by many others, including the Nobel Laureates Brown and Goldstein (Figure 1). After his death Michael Brown wrote "When we entered the field we found him to be one of a very small number of linear thinkers. The rest were running around in circles. We held him in the highest regard."

American Pioneers

Inherited disorders of lipid metabolism such as FH were also the object of considerable attention during the 1950s and 1960s from Donald Fredrickson at the US National Institutes of Health (NIH) in Bethesda, Maryland. He joined the staff there in 1953 and published his first paper on lipids the following year. He later recalled attending a symposium in 1957 in New Orleans with Ancel Keys, Alistair ("Fats") Frazer and John Youmans,

Dean of Vanderbilt University. The last-named took them to a bar in the French Quarter, where they ran up a large bill buying watered-down drinks for the bar girls. Youmans had apparently been a jazz trumpeter in the city in his youth, so he knew the ropes and led them out without paying, pursued by the bartenders and girls.[17]

Fredrickson's research focused on the role of lipoproteins in transporting lipids in plasma and the familial disorders characterized by lipoprotein abnormalities in patients referred to the NIH.

At the beginning of 1967, Fredrickson, Levy, and Lees published a multipart paper in the *New England Journal of Medicine*, which described the phenotypic classification (clinical and biochemical expression) of five different types of hyperlipoproteinaemia[18] and thereby revolutionized the attitude of clinicians to lipids. Among those infected with enthusiasm were two young interns, Goldstein and Brown, at the Mass General in Boston. I was a research fellow there at that time, and I can still recall the excitement generated by Fredrickson *et al.*'s paper. Joe Goldstein subsequently looked after Fredrickson's patients when he was a clinical associate at the NIH, and it was this experience that stimulated his interest in FH, an interest he communicated to Mike Brown. Their subsequent scientific collaboration at the University of Texas Southwestern Medical School in Dallas resulted in their Nobel Prize-winning discovery of the LDL receptor and the role played by genetic mutations of the latter in causing FH.[19] Fredrickson's colleague at the NIH, Bob Levy, had earlier shown that the fractional rate of turnover of ^{125}I-labelled LDL was reduced in FH patients,[20] implying the existence of an *in vivo* catabolic defect, and the underlying deficiency of LDL receptors that was responsible was revealed by Goldstein and Brown's *in vitro* studies.

The 1970s were halcyon years for clinicians and biochemists interested in lipids, but, as will become apparent later, the relevance of advances in lipid research to atherosclerosis and coronary disease was still disputed by some cardiologists, who were accused at the time of practising "paleocardiology," as distinct from "neocardiology."[21]

Fredrickson was appointed Director of the National Heart Institute in 1966 and became the director of the NIH in 1975. He later summarized the progress which occurred between 1950 and 1975 as a Bethesda-driven "climb to base camp" that preceded the conjunction of molecular biology with the research on lipoproteins and disorders thereof.[22] His inspiration and leadership during that early phase of exploration were an essential preliminary to the successful scaling of scientific peaks by others, such as Goldstein and Brown. It would be hard to overestimate the influence he exerted on lipid research and research workers throughout the world during that remarkable era of progress. By differentiating between the phenotypes of the various types of lipoprotein disorder, Fredrickson stimulated the search for the pathological mechanisms responsible and thereby set the stage for the discovery of the underlying gene defects, currently a topic of intense research activity throughout the world.

References

1. Somerville J. The master's legacy: The first Paul Wood lecture. *Heart* 1998;**80**:612–19.
2. Obituary: Edward Peter Sharpey-Schafer. *Br Heart J* 1964;**26**:430–2.
3. Oliver M. Cholesterol, atherosclerosis and coronary disease in the UK, 1950–2000. In Reynolds LA, Tansey EM (eds.), *Wellcome Witnesses to Twentieth Century Medicine*, Vol. 27, 2006, p. 4.
4. Oliver M. Cholesterol, atherosclerosis and coronary disease in the UK, 1950–2000. In Reynolds LA, Tansey EM (eds.), *Wellcome Witnesses to Twentieth Century Medicine*, Vol. 27, 2006, p. 7.
5. Oliver MF, Boyd GS. The plasma lipids in coronary artery disease. *Br Heart J* 1953;**15**:387–92.
6. Oliver MF, Boyd GS. Serum lipoprotein patterns in coronary sclerosis and associated conditions. *Br Heart J* 1955;**17**:299–302.
7. Oliver MF, Boyd GS. Influence of reduction of serum lipids on prognosis of coronary artery diseases — a five-year study using oestrogen. *Lancet* 1961;**ii**:499–505.
8. Bronte-Stewart B. The effect of dietary fats on the blood lipids and their relation to ischaemic heart disease. *Br Med Bull* 1958;**14**:243–52.
9. Pappworth MH. *Human Guinea Pigs: Experimentation on Man.* London: Beacon Press, 1968.
10. Morris JN, Heady JA, Raffle PA, Roberts CG, Parks JW. Coronary heart-disease and physical activity of work. *Lancet* 1953;**265**:1053–7.
11. Morris JN, Heady JA, Raffle PA, Roberts CG, Parks JW. Coronary heart-disease and physical activity of work. *Lancet* 1953;**265**:1111–20.

12. Morris J. Cholesterol, atherosclerosis and coronary disease in the UK, 1950–2000. In Reynolds LA, Tansey EM (eds.), *Wellcome Witnesses to Twentieth Century Medicine*, Vol. 27, 2006, p. 42.
13. Frazer AC. Lipid metabolism: Introduction. *Br Med Bull* 1958;**14**:197–200.
14. Myant NB. Introduction. Cholesterol, atherosclerosis and coronary disease in the UK, 1950- 2000. In Reynolds LA, Tansey EM (eds.), *Wellcome Witnesses to Twentieth Century Medicine*, Vol. 27, 2006, p. xxiii.
15. Müller C. Angina pectoris in hereditary xanthomatosis. *Arch Intern Med* 1939;**64**:675–700.
16. Myant NB. The regulation of cholesterol metabolism as related to familial hypercholesterolaemia. *Sci Basis Med Annu Rev* 1970; Chapter XIV:230–59.
17. http://profiles.nlm.nih.gov/FF/B/B/L/G/_/ffbblg.txt.
18. Fredrickson DS, Levy RI, Lees RS. Fat transport in lipoproteins — an integrated approach to mechanisms and disorders. *N Engl J Med* 1967;**276**: 34–42, 94–103, 148–56, 215–25, 273–81.
19. Goldstein JL, Brown MS. Familial hypercholesterolemia: Identification of a defect in the regulation of 3-hydroxy-3-methylglutaryl coenzyme A reductase activity associated with overproduction of cholesterol. *Proc Natl Acad Sci USA* 1973;**70**:2804–8.
20. Langer T, Strober W, Levy RI. The metabolism of low density lipoprotein in familial type II hyperlipoproteinemia. *J Clin Invest* 1972;**51**:1528–36.
21. Carruthers M, Taggart P. Paleocardiology and neocardiology. *Am Heart J* 1974;**88**:1–6.
22. Fredrickson DS. Phenotyping. On reaching base camp (1950–1975). *Circulation* 1993;**87**(Suppl 4):III1–15.

8 Sir John McMichael's Anti-Cholesterol Campaign

John McMichael

It must be obvious by now that not all cardiologists accepted the lipid hypothesis of atherosclerosis, namely that raised levels of cholesterol in the blood result in the accumulation of cholesterol in the walls of arteries, thereby narrowing them and causing heart attacks. Chief among the doubters in Britain was Sir John McMichael, once described as the greatest clinical scientist of his generation. He directed the Department of Medicine at the Hammersmith from 1946 to 1966, and to those of us who worked under him he was an Olympian figure akin to "M" in the James Bond films, evoking in equal measure fear and respect, admiration and affection. He himself attributed the success of the department to the inspired choice of staff made by his predecessor Francis Frazer in pre-war years, when the Postgraduate Medical School was founded. These included Paul Wood, Peter Sharpey-Schafer, and many other outstanding clinical research workers, including McMichael himself.

After the war, however, McMichael's ability to create an atmosphere of enthusiasm, constructive criticism, and cooperation was such that the best young research workers were attracted by the reputations of the people working there, and this earned worldwide recognition for the Hammersmith as the best place for UK and Commonwealth graduates to do their postgraduate medical training.[1] At the instigation of Australian postgraduates, one of the first places in London where imported Foster's lager was available was the doctors' bar (now defunct) that was adjacent to the aptly named Commonwealth Building at the Hammersmith; in those days most postgraduates came from Australia, Canada, New Zealand, and South Africa.

Many members of McMichael's department went on to fill Chairs elsewhere, such as Sheila Sherlock (later a Dame) at the Royal Free Hospital, Malcolm Milne at the Westminster Hospital, both of whom became Fellows of the Royal Society, and Peter Sharpey-Schafer at St. Thomas's. Those of us who attended the weekly staff round that McMichael chaired on Wednesday mornings in the Wolfson Building will recall his gentle handling of young presenters of cases, which could be a nerve-wracking occasion for the uninitiated. Nerve-wracking not only for juniors but also for more senior individuals such as the visiting consultant neurologist from the West End Hospital for Nervous Diseases, who had an attack of stress-induced dysphasia when invited to comment on a case. He started off by saying "Our policy at the Nervous Hospital for West End Diseases is ..." whereupon the rest of his sentence was drowned out by peals of laughter from the audience, including its chairman!

Following his departure from the Hammersmith in 1966, McMichael became Director of the British Postgraduate Medical Federation and continued to influence postgraduate medical training for several years. Numerous honours and awards were bestowed upon him, including Fellowship of the Royal Society and a knighthood (Figure 1). In 1975, he gave the Harveian Oration at the Royal College of Physicians and during his discourse he commented "Resistance to change is far from unknown among great scientists," citing Virchow's rejection of Koch's pioneering work.[2] Ironically, this statement was prophetic of his own attitude to the lipid hypothesis in subsequent years.

Retired but not Quietly

In 1973, 3 years after he retired from the British Postgraduate Medical Federation and long after his departure from the Hammersmith, McMichael started a campaign against those who believed that diet and exercise played a role in the aetiology of coronary heart disease. In the first of several letters to *The Lancet* from his house in North Square, Hampstead, he criticized the International Society of Cardiology for stating that an increased intake of cholesterol and fat is a prerequisite for the development of atherosclerosis, and took issue with data showing that exercise has a protective effect.[3] With some reluctance, since I was working in the

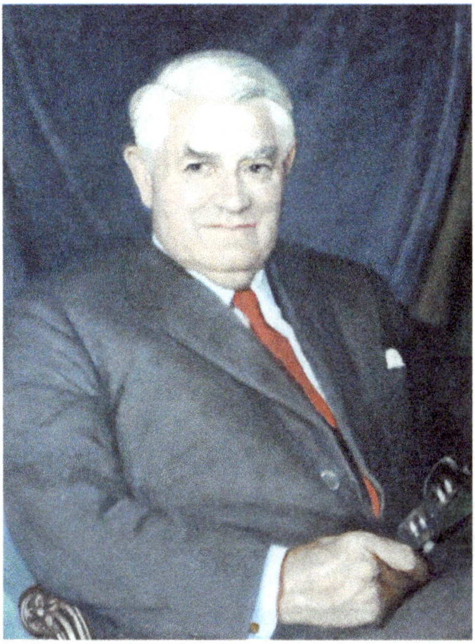

Figure 1. Portrait of Sir John McMichael (1904–1993) painted by Sir William Hutchison in 1968.

department he had once directed and where he had given me my first job 11 years previously, I rebutted McMichael's arguments and suggested that cardiologists and those involved in research into atherosclerosis should start a constructive dialogue.[4] This proposal fell on deaf ears and led me to cite Medawar's story of the famous wit Sydney Smith who, when he came upon two housewives arguing from windows on opposite sides of a street in Edinburgh, commented "They can never agree for they are arguing from different premises."

Two years later, McMichael returned to the fray to criticize the recommendations of a joint working party of the Royal College of Physicians and the British Cardiac Society on the Prevention of Coronary Disease, which endorsed the policy of reducing saturated fat intake to lower serum cholesterol.[5] He reiterated his conviction that this measure would have little effect on the incidence of coronary disease and concluded that "it is better to trust to luck than to foster neurosis by pretence that we can save lives by interfering with life habits." The Chairman of the Joint Working Party, Gerry Shaper, responded that the measures recommended in the report had a reasonable hope of conferring benefit, and none had a cost that approached the cost of inaction.[6] McMichael was unimpressed and again criticized the report for its simplistic dietetic advice and the manner in which its views were publicized by the Department of Health, which had sent a copy to every doctor.[7] Further support for the report came from John Goodwin, who had been a member of McMichael's department from its early days. He had instigated the joint working party when he was president of the British Cardiac Society and defended the advice it gave to the medical profession aimed at preventing coronary disease.[8]

McMichael then turned his attention to the recently published results of the Whitehall Study and questioned whether the correlation of raised cholesterol with coronary risk in patients with angina or an abnormal ECG might be a consequence of their heart disease rather than a cause, as Paul Wood had suggested many years previously.[9] This comment, like many of McMichael's criticisms pertaining to lipids and epidemiology, was scientifically naïve in ignoring the fact that hypercholesterolaemia is present from birth in FH patients, long before they develop heart disease, but his past achievements and considerable reputation lent credence to his arguments and ensured that they were well publicized.

European Society for Clinical Investigation Debate

The chance to put all these arguments to the test came in 1977 when the European Society for Clinical Investigation (ESCI) held a "Controversy in medicine" debate at its annual meeting in Rotterdam. The motion to be debated was "That modification of serum lipids by dietary and/or other means will influence the incidence of, or mortality from, coronary heart disease" and was chaired by Hermon Dowling. In favour of the motion were Lars Carlson from Stockholm, Shlomo Eisenberg from Jerusalem, and myself. Lars was the premier clinical lipidologist in Europe at the time while Shlomo had established a major reputation as a result of the research he had carried out with Levy at the NIH. Against the motion were Sir John

McMichael and Professors Paul Astrup and Christian Crone, both from Copenhagen.

The proponents of the motion put forward a tripartite case for there being a causal association between hyperlipidaemia and coronary disease and postulated that reversal of the former would reduce the incidence of the latter. This was based on three lines of scientific evidence, epidemiological, experimental and clinical, which we presented in an orthodox manner. The case against the motion was then put by Christian Crone, who showed two slides. The first was a photograph of a sleek, well-groomed rat, which, he said, had been fed on butter from birth, while the second showed a malnourished rodent with dull, moulting fur, which, he claimed, had been fed on corn oil throughout its short life. The audience dissolved into fits of laughter, and Crone's debating ploy ensured that the motion was lost, much to McMichael's delight and our discomfort.

The following year the results of the WHO trial of the lipid-lowering drug clofibrate were published, which showed an increase in non-cardiovascular causes of death in those in the trial who were on the drug. McMichael was not slow to capitalize on this finding, and in January 1979 he published a paper in the *British Medical Journal* entitled "Fats and atheroma: An inquest."[10] In this, he alluded to the negative results of some of the early diet trials as casting doubt on the role of cholesterol in atherosclerosis, and he pointed out the potential dangers of lowering blood levels by polyunsaturated fats and clofibrate, namely cancer of the colon and gallstones, respectively. He concluded that official medical endorsement of these cholesterol-reducing measures should be withdrawn. In a similar paper published later that year, he characterized the campaign to substitute polyunsaturated for saturated fats as a "quite unwarranted extension of hope over experience."[11]

Taking a leaf out of McMichael's tactics in the Rotterdam debate and satirizing his previous use of the inquest theme, I published a letter in the *Acta Medica Scandinavica* which parodied Mark Antony's funeral oration in *Julius Caesar.*[12]

> This commenced:
>
> Friends, clinicians, colleagues, lend me your eyes;
> I come to bury the Lipid Hypothesis, not to praise it.

And ended:

My heart is in the coffin there with the Lipid Hypothesis,
And atheroma must regress before it come back to life.

Attempts to Demonstrate Regression of Atherosclerosis

Demonstrating regression of atheroma, that is to say the movement of cholesterol out of diseased arteries consequent upon therapeutic reductions in plasma cholesterol levels, would strengthen the case for the lipid hypothesis. This was not just wishful thinking because for the previous 5 years my colleagues and I had continued to treat a small number of patients with FH with plasma exchange, mainly homozygotes (2 mutant alleles) and severely affected heterozygotes (1 mutant allele). Many of the former had atherosclerotic involvement of the aortic root and valve, whereas the latter usually had three-vessel coronary artery disease. Interestingly, the aortic lesion in homozygotes is almost identical to that demonstrated by Anitschkow in cholesterol-fed rabbits in 1913.[13] He went on to show regression of their atherosclerosis after cholesterol feeding was discontinued and their very high cholesterol levels had returned to normal on their usual diet. Unfortunately, it is not so easy to lower the very high cholesterol levels that characterise homozygous FH in humans.

The significance of Anitschkow's work led Steinberg to describe him as the founding father of the lipid hypothesis of atherosclerosis,[14] a scientist who he considered was worthy of a Nobel Prize and who was the inspiration for much of his own research. The esteem in which Steinberg himself was held and the importance of his research into atherosclerosis were highlighted after his death in a tribute to him in the *Proceedings of the National Academy of Sciences USA*, of which he was a member.[15] His diminutive stature belied the size of his intellect and the warmth of his relationships with friends and colleagues who had earned his respect.

The first evidence of benefit from plasma exchange came after 6 months, with a diminution in the size of cutaneous xanthomas (yellowish accumulations of cholesterol in the skin) in our homozygotes. Achilles tendon xanthomas took years rather than months but these too started to shrink in size. What we now needed to know was whether similar changes were occurring in the aorta and coronary arteries.

Coronary angiography at the Hammersmith in the 1970s was undertaken by radiologists, not by cardiologists, so Celia Oakley and I enlisted the help of Robert Steiner and Maurice Raphael to study our FH patients. They performed serial angiography using the old-fashioned equipment then in use. Since the X-ray tube was fixed, taking oblique and lateral views meant tilting the patient on the metal stretcher, all the while keeping the cardiac catheter in place and preventing it from wedging in the ostium (mouth) of the coronary artery, which was not an easy task. By this means and by measuring the gradient across the aortic valve, we were able to show that 2–3 years of plasma exchange slowed the rate of progression of atherosclerosis in homozygotes and induced actual regression in some heterozygotes, in whom we could achieve much lower cholesterol levels than in homozygotes. Publication of our angiographic results in 1980 provided preliminary evidence, albeit uncontrolled, that cholesterol-lowering was beneficial in patients with severe, genetically determined hypercholesterolaemia.[16]

Early Prevention Trials

With regard to the role of lifestyle changes in preventing coronary heart disease, derided by McMichael, the publication in 1981 of the Oslo 5-years-trial of dietary and anti-smoking measures demonstrated a 45% reduction in coronary events in high-risk Norwegian men. However, it was unclear to what extent this reflected the 13% reduction in serum cholesterol or the 45% decrease in smoking.[17] The relevance of lowering cholesterol, specifically lowering LDL cholesterol, the major carrier of cholesterol in plasma, gained further support from the publication in 1984 of the results of the LRC Primary Prevention Trial of cholestyramine.[18] This drug works by reducing reabsorption of bile acids, which are the breakdown products of cholesterol. This results in an increased rate of conversion of cholesterol into bile acids and thereby lowers the amount of cholesterol available for transport by LDL in the blood stream. This multi-million dollar endeavour was masterminded by Bob Levy (Figure 2) at the NIH, and the 19% reduction in coronary events in cholestyramine-treated subjects compared with those

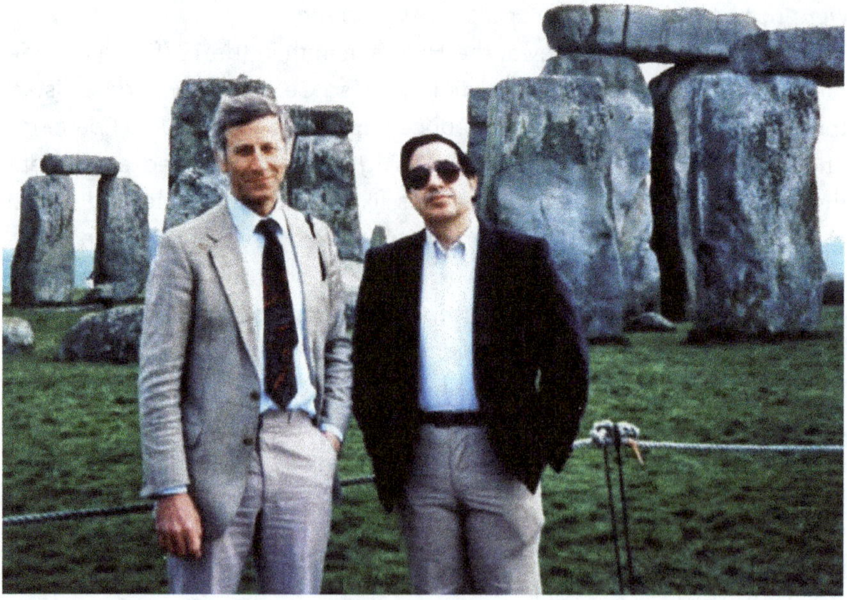

Figure 2. The author with Bob Levy (1937–2001) at Stonehenge.

on placebo convinced lipidologists, if not cardiologists, that cholesterol lowering was worthwhile. Had the outcome been negative, this would have had a disastrous impact on the future development of lipid-lowering drugs.

A number of other trials subsequently showed similar results, including one by Buchwald *et al.* that used the surgical procedure of partial ileal bypass to induce bile acid malabsorption by an analogous but more effective mechanism than cholestyramine and thus lowered LDL to an even greater extent.[19] After 10 years of follow-up there was less angiographic progression of coronary atherosclerosis and fewer coronary events in those who had undergone partial ileal bypass. Hence, by 1990 the validity of the lipid hypothesis had received substantial support, these trials having helped it to "come back to life."

Demise of an Icon

In 1985, a special staff round chaired by Keith Peters was held at Hammersmith to celebrate Sir John McMichael's 80th birthday. Sadly, he had by then sustained a severe stroke and was confined to a wheelchair. I presented one of the cases, a patient with severe hyperlipidaemia who had responded well to lipid-lowering therapy. Sir John nodded and smiled benignly, but his aphasia made it impossible to know whether he had changed his mind about cholesterol. It seemed improbable but not impossible, for in his Harveian Oration he had quoted a passage from William Harvey's *De Motu Cordis*: "Studious good and honest men do not think it degrading to alter their view if truth and a public demonstration so persuade them ..."

After he died in 1993, a service of thanksgiving was held for him at St. Columba's Church of Scotland in London. It was packed with Hammersmith staff, past and present, united in paying tribute to a great man. As Chris Booth said in his obituary,[20] McMichael had created a clinical research environment, unique in Britain at that time, of free discussion and debate in which all, at whatever level of seniority, might join. His opposition to the lipid hypothesis may in part have reflected an ageing man's reaction against the need to acquire sufficient biochemical knowledge to comprehend it fully. Whether or not that was so, the vigour with which he contested its validity helped ensure that proof of the hypothesis, when it eventually came, was based on the hard evidence he had long demanded. Although the errors that men publish live after them, the good that John McMichael did at the Hammersmith has also survived and, contradicting Shakespeare, was not interred with his bones.

References

1. Farewell at Hammersmith. *Br Med J* 1966;**2**:320.
2. McMichael J. *A Transition in Cardiology: The Mackenzie–Lewis Era*. The Harveian Oration of 1975. London: Royal College of Physicians, 1976.
3. McMichael J. Diet and exercise in coronary heart-disease [Letter]. *Lancet* 1974;**1**:1340–1.
4. Thompson G. Diet and coronary heart-disease [Letter]. *Lancet* 1974;**13**:102.
5. McMichael J. Prevention of coronary heart-disease [Letter]. *Lancet* 1976;**2**:569.
6. Shaper G. Prevention of coronary heart-disease [Letter]. *Lancet* 1976;**2**: 1203–4.
7. McMichael J. Prevention of coronary heart-disease. *Lancet* 1976;**2**:1350–1.
8. Goodwin JF. Preventing coronary heart-disease [Letter]. *Lancet* 1977;**1**:302.

9. McMichael J. Risk factors in coronary heart-disease [Letter]. *Lancet* 1977;**1**:304.
10. McMichael J. Fats and atheroma: An inquest. *Br Med J* 1979;**1**:173–5.
11. McMichael J. Fats and arterial disease. *Am Heart J* 1979;**98**:409–12.
12. Thompson G. The lipid hypothesis [Letter]. *Acta Med Scand* 1980;**208**:341–2.
13. Thompson GR. Atherosclerosis in cholesterol-fed rabbits and in homozygous and heterozygous LDL receptor-deficient humans. *Atherosclerosis* 2018;**276**:148–54.
14. Steinberg D. Nikolai Anitschkow: The birth of the lipid hypothesis of atherosclerosis and coronary heart disease. In Thompson G (ed.), *Pioneers of Medicine without a Nobel Prize*, Imperial College Press, London, 2014, pp. 23–39.
15. Glass CK, Witzum JL. Daniel Steinberg, 1922–2015. *Proc Nat Acad Sci USA* 2015;**112**:9791–92.
16. Thompson GR, Myant NB, Kilpatrick D, Oakley CM, Raphael MJ, Steiner RE. Assessment of long-term plasma exchange for familial hypercholesterolaemia. *Br Heart J* 1980;**43**:680–8.
17. Hjermann I, Holme I, Velve Byre K, Leren P. Effect of diet and smoking intervention on the incidence of coronary heart disease. Report from the Oslo study group of a randomised trial in healthy men. *Lancet* 1981;**ii**:1303–10.
18. Lipid Research Clinics Program. The Lipid Research Clinics Coronary Primary Prevention Trial results. 1. Reduction in incidence of coronary heart disease. *JAMA* 1984;**251**:351–64.
19. Buchwald H, Varco RL, Matts JP *et al.* Effect of partial ileal bypass surgery on mortality and morbidity from coronary heart disease in patients with hypercholestrolemia. *N Eng J Med* 1990;**323**:945–55.
20. Booth C. Sir John McMichael [Obituary]. *Lancet* 1993;**341**:686.

9 Should Every Cow Carry a Government Health Warning?

Tony Mitchell

Sir John McMichael was not the only heavyweight opponent of the lipid hypothesis in Britain. One of the keenest minds and sharpest tongues belonged to JRA (Tony) Mitchell, the foundation Professor of Medicine at Nottingham University from 1967 until his retirement in 1990. He died the following year from a pulmonary embolus, which was ironic in that clotting was one of his main scientific interests. His early research was performed in the department of the Regius Professor of Medicine at Oxford, where he and Colin Schwartz studied the pathology of atherosclerosis. In a book they published on the subject, they proposed that turbulent blood flow at sites of arterial branching caused platelets to coalesce and form mural thrombi (clots), resulting in the formation of raised plaques on the arterial intima.[1] This concept was in keeping with the Duguid theory that regarded thrombosis as the cause rather than the consequence of atherosclerosis, in contrast to the lipid hypothesis the validity of which Mitchell constantly questioned. From the mid-1960s onwards, he and his collaborators turned their attention to platelet structure and function, initially in Oxford and then in Nottingham. This led them to study factors influencing platelet behaviour and to undertake clinical trials with anti-platelet drugs in patients with myocardial infarction.

COMA

Tony Mitchell was a member of the first COMA of diet and coronary heart disease, which published its recommendations in 1974.[2] Other members of the committee included Oliver, Morris, and Yudkin, and Mitchell later gave a revealing account of the manner in which its deliberations were conducted.[3] He described the agreed brief as being to establish whether there was a link between nutrition and cardiovascular disease and, if so, to determine whether modifying the identified risk factor conferred benefit on the individual or community. After many meetings and draft reports, the committee was able to conclude that ischaemic heart disease was multifactorial in origin and that some of the factors involved were dietary in nature but that no single one was predominantly responsible. It also agreed that changes in diet could reduce serum lipids but that there was no certainty that their reduction would decrease susceptibility to heart disease. The majority of members of the panel accepted the evidence that the death rate from ischaemic heart disease correlated with the saturated fat content of the diet and therefore recommended that the amount of saturated fat in the diet should be reduced. A minority of the members disagreed with this conclusion and felt that this recommendation went beyond the evidence available. However, apart from Yudkin, whose dissent has already been noted, they agreed to support the corporate viewpoint, albeit reluctantly as far as Mitchell was concerned because he undoubtedly belonged to the minority camp on this issue (Figure 1).

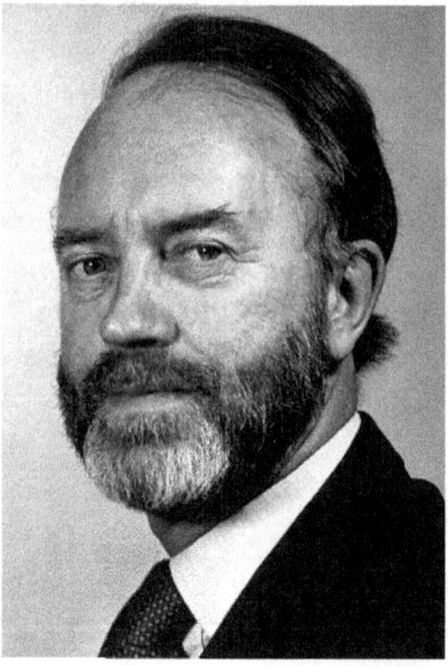

Figure 1. Tony Mitchell (1928–1991) (photograph by courtesy of Professor John Hampton).

In 1984, a second COMA report was published on diet in relation to cardiovascular disease.[4] Tony Mitchell and Michael Oliver were again members of the committee, but it now had several newcomers and on this occasion the recommendations regarding the need to reduce the saturated fat content of the diet and to increase its ratio of polyunsaturated to saturated fat were far more specific than those made 10 years previously. Nine of the ten members of the panel concluded that the incidence of coronary heart disease would be reduced by such measures, although they acknowledged that the evidence fell short of proof. The tenth member, who was not named but was undoubtedly Mitchell,[5] believed that the evidence was insufficient to support that conclusion but considered that reducing dietary fat intake might help prevent obesity.

Doubts About Diet and Coronary Disease

Mitchell amplified his doubts in an editorial review published the same year as the second COMA report.[6] He prefaced it by quoting HL Mencken, "There's always an easy solution to every human problem — neat, plausible and wrong," and went on to question which of the beliefs about diet and coronary disease, then current, would not only be discarded but also derided by the year 2000. He listed them as follows:

- Coronary heart disease is caused by atherosclerosis.
- Atherosclerotic plaques are cholesterol deposits in artery walls.
- Atherosclerosis can be produced in animals by lipid feeding.
- A high serum cholesterol is a risk marker for coronary disease.
- Dietary lipids determine serum cholesterol.

He went on to point out that if these statements were true, two further ones followed:

- Dietary lipids cause coronary heart disease.
- Dietary modifications will prevent coronary heart disease.

Mitchell then put his head on the block by stating that as far as he was concerned most of these beliefs were untrue or irrelevant. It is now apparent that he was wrong on virtually every count, although this was not quite so obvious at the time, especially regarding the last statement in that the evidence from diet trials was at best equivocal.

Mitchell's approach to prevention in the clinic was to tell his patients to stop smoking but to say nothing on issues such as diet. He attributed to Oliver a similarly cautious approach, which led them, he said, to be labelled "the abominable no-men" by "cholesterol evangelists." His own attitude to the latter was equally pejorative. For example, the title of one of his lectures was "Should every cow carry a government health warning?"[7] while his publications had titles such as "Diet and arterial disease — the myths and the realities"[8] and "What constitutes evidence on the dietary prevention of coronary heart disease? Cosy beliefs or harsh facts?"[6] He ended the latter editorial as he had started it, by quoting HL Mencken: "The most costly of all follies is to believe passionately in the palpably-not-true." Or is it even more costly to passionately deny, as he did, what turns out later to be palpably true?

During the late 1970s and early 1980s, McMichael and Mitchell voiced their opposition to the lipid hypothesis in unequivocal terms whereas Oliver adopted an ambivalent attitude. For example, in an editorial in 1976, he stated, "the view that raised plasma cholesterol is per se a cause of coronary heart disease is untenable," but then went on to encourage people to reduce their saturated fat intake so as to reduce their risk of coronary heart disease, while omitting to mention that this would result in a decrease in plasma cholesterol.[9] All three were influential cardiologists and their views undoubtedly affected clinical attitudes among their peers.

Mitchell maintained his sceptical attitude to the evidence relating to the prevention of coronary disease right up until his retirement in 1990. By then, the results of the early lipid-lowering drug trials were available, including the LRC Coronary Primary Prevention trial, which he dismissed as an extravagant waste of money.[10] Like McMichael, he was consistent in his demand for unequivocal proof but like him he died before it became available.

Despite his "Dr No" image among supporters of the lipid hypothesis, Tony Mitchell had many positive qualities and was regarded as the major architect of Nottingham's success as a medical school and centre of scientific excellence.[7] At one stage, there was a move to persuade him to stand for the presidency of the Royal College of Physicians, but he refused on the grounds that becoming the president would force him to change himself more than he could change the college. His strongly held principles meant that he was unwilling to compromise with NHS reforms during the 1980s, and this led him to take early retirement. He was an excellent speaker, discussant, and chairman and filled the latter role with distinction for several years in the Atherosclerosis Discussion Group (ADG), which subsequently became the British Atherosclerosis Society.

The ADG and the British Atherosclerosis Society

The origins of the ADG go back to 1957, when Michael Oliver, working in Edinburgh, wrote to John French at the Dunn School of Pathology in Oxford, expressing concern that there was no organization in Britain interested in the relationship of lipid metabolism, blood flow, and platelets to experimental atherosclerosis. French invited Oliver to come to Oxford to meet his boss, Sir Howard Florey, who, having won the Nobel Prize for his work on penicillin, had now become interested in vascular pathology. At their meeting, Florey told French to make a list of those working in the field of atherosclerosis and asked Oliver to raise enough money to hold an inaugural meeting. With the help of Dr "Cuth" Cuthbertson at Glaxo, Oliver raised the required £250 and French produced a list of people to invite. The first meeting of the new group, comprising 27 members, was held in the autumn of 1958 at the old MRC headquarters in London, the topic being "Interrelationships of dietary fat, blood lipids, and atherosclerosis." Lord Florey, as he became, was the first Chairman and Michael Oliver the first Secretary of the ADG, later succeeded by John French. Florey stipulated that there must be an equal time allocated for discussion as for presentation. Hence, the name Atherosclerosis Discussion Group.

The ADG initially consisted mainly of pathologists plus a few biochemists, cardiologists, and people interested in lipid metabolism and blood coagulation. Its membership was limited to 50 and meetings were held twice a year, in the spring and the autumn, initially at the Ciba Foundation in London or at one of the Oxford colleges. In later years, the spring meetings were always held in Oxford, thanks to John Hampton, who, while secretary of the ADG, persuaded Hugh Sinclair, who had been his tutor at Magdalen College, to play host there. The autumn ones were held at Jesus College, Cambridge, where Austin Gresham, the Professor of Pathology, was a Fellow.

The meetings lived up to the group's name, and discussion took up as much if not more time than the presentation of data. The facilities were far from luxurious, the heating being non-existent at Magdalen, and the projection equipment was primitive. Despite this, the multidisciplinary mix of the various members and their guests in cramped surroundings resulted in stimulating, close-quarter exchanges between people with opposing views, Tony Mitchell being in his element on these occasions. Afterwards, protagonists and antagonists chatted amicably over a glass or two of sherry before dining in the hall of the college where the meeting was held.

In 1975, only 3 of the 47 members were women, 2 of whom were pathologists, namely Helen Payling Wright, one of the founder members, and Elspeth Smith, also a founder member and the first to show a relationship between the concentration of LDL in the plasma and the arterial wall.[11] The third was the geneticist Joan Slack, best known for quantifying the risk of coronary disease in FH.[12] This bias persisted and Anne Soutar has recalled how few women there still were when she was elected to the ADG, many years later.[13] Yet, despite its elitist nature and distinguished membership, the group as a whole failed to influence medical opinion in Britain regarding the cholesterol controversy as much as it might have done. This may have been because the views of its members on the matter were divided, although there were some, such as Mitchell and Oliver, who were certainly not shy of voicing their opinions in public.

Inevitably, the ADG lost some of its intimacy when its membership expanded and it became the British Atherosclerosis Society (BAS) in 1998, a change that I initiated during my tenure as its Chairman. However, the emphasis on time for discussion has been preserved, as has the tradition of alternating meetings between Oxford and Cambridge. John French died in 1970, and his influence on the field of atherosclerosis research is commemorated with the John French Memorial Lecture, which is given annually at the spring meeting. French's remarkable insight into the pathology of atherosclerosis is illustrated by the observation he made over 60 years ago that the lipid composition of the tissue fluid was responsible for the overall severity of tissue changes, whereas the main determinant of clinical events was thrombosis.[14]

Hugh Sinclair

In an analogous manner, the Hugh Sinclair Memorial Lecture is given at each autumn meeting in recognition of Sinclair's pioneering work on the nutritional aspects of atherosclerosis. He was interested in the role of diet but he did not subscribe to the traditional view that a high fat diet caused high serum cholesterol, which caused atherosclerosis, which caused coronary disease. His opposition was based on his knowledge of Eskimos, whose fat intake was extremely high but in whom coronary disease was uncommon. Since most of their fat is polyunsaturated Sinclair proposed that it was the relative deficiency of essential (polyunsaturated) fatty acids in Western diets that was atherogenic, rather than the high intake of total fat.[15] He went on to postulate that a high ratio of non-essential to essential fatty acids in the diet promoted fatty streaks in the arterial wall by increasing the proportion of cholesterol esterified with oleic acid (a non-essential fatty acid with one double bond) at the expense of linoleic acid (an essential fatty acid with two double bonds).[16]

Sinclair's interest in the effects of the Eskimo diet was such that he lived for 3 months on food derived entirely from marine sources, consisting mainly of seal meat. He then analysed the resulting changes in the fatty acid composition of his plasma lipids, platelets, and various tissues obtained by biopsy, including a testicular biopsy.[17] However, his bleeding time was so prolonged that the liver biopsy he requested was ruled out as too dangerous! Although Sinclair's theory that atherosclerosis was a form of essential fatty acid deficiency was not substantiated by the evidence, his belief in the benefits of ω3 fatty acids and the harmful effects of trans-fatty acids resulting from hydrogenation of oils are now widely accepted. One of Hugh's endearing eccentricities was to send his friends Christmas greetings in the form of rhyming verse. An example of this was a chorus to be sung to the tune of Auld Lang Syne: "So let us eat these fats much more, ω6 and 3, we'll take a cup of palm oil for, our platelets will be free!" The problem with this sentiment is that eating "much more" ω3 fatty acids caused the platelet deficiency that Hugh sustained while he was on his seal diet, a case of having too much of a good thing.

Much of what the ADG used to debate with such energy is now old hat, and the emphasis has shifted to the cell biology of the arterial wall and atheromatous plaques. For example, a recent BAS meeting included topics such as "Using transcriptomics to understand macrophage function in human atherosclerotic plaques," "Global Epigenetics of Atherosclerotic Smooth Muscle cells," and "Matrix Metalloproteinase regulation of vulnerable plaques." Nevertheless, the Society continues to provide a means of communication between clinicians and basic scientists doing research on various aspects of atherosclerosis. It thereby perpetuates the aims and objectives of its founders, some of whom were present at its 100th meeting, which was celebrated in September 2008 at Queen's College, Cambridge (Figure 2).

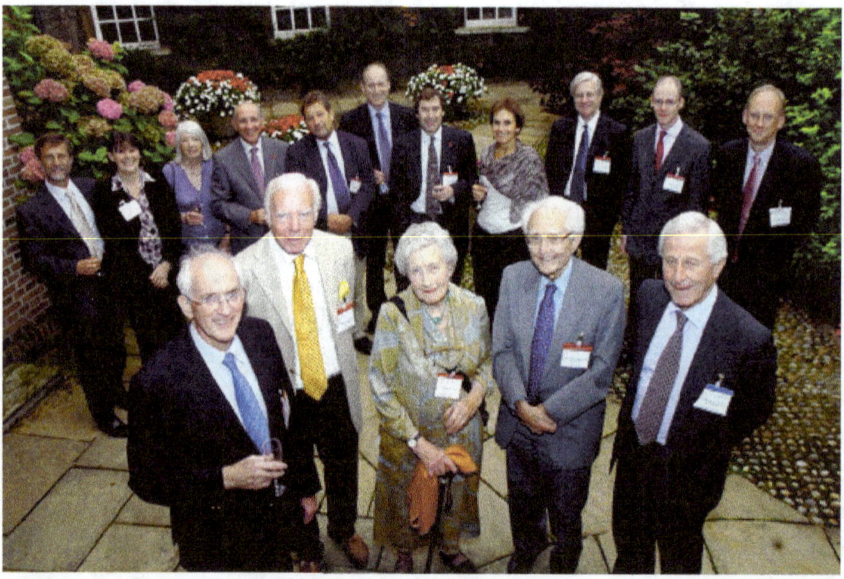

Figure 2. Past and present officers of the British Atherosclerosis Society in 2008. Back row: Steve Humphries; Sarah Jane George; Anne Soutar; Peter Weissberg; Tom Sanders; Dorian Haskard; Jeremy Pearson; Philippa Talmud; Paul Miller; Keith Channon; and Chris Newman. Front row: John Hampton; Michael Oliver (1925–2015); Elspeth Smith (1923–2017); Gustaf Born (1921–2018); and the Author (reproduced by permission of the British Atherosclerosis Society).

References

1. Mitchell JRA, Schwartz CJ. *Arterial Disease*. Oxford: Blackwell Scientific, 1965.
2. Department of Health and Social Security. Report on Health and Society Subjects. 7. *Diet and Coronary Heart Disease*. Report of the Advisory Panel of the Committee on Medical Aspects of Food Policy (Nutrition) on diet in relation to Cardiovascular and Cerebrovascular Disease. London: HMSO, 1974.
3. Mitchell JRA. Diet and coronary heart disease — a British point of view. *Adv Exp Med Biol* 1977;**82**:823–7.
4. Department of Health and Social Security. Report on Health and Society Subjects. 28. *Diet and Cardiovascular Disease*. Committee on Medical Aspects of Food Policy. Report of the Panel on Diet in Relation to Cardiovascular Disease. London: HMSO, 1984.
5. Sanders TAB. Cholesterol, atherosclerosis and coronary disease in the UK, 1950-2000. In Reynolds LA, Tansey EM (eds.), *Wellcome Witnesses to Twentieth Century Medicine*, Vol. 27, 2006, p. 62.
6. Mitchell JRA. What constitutes evidence on the dietary prevention of coronary heart disease? Cosy beliefs or harsh facts? *Int J Cardiol* 1984;**5**:287–98.
7. Mitchell JRA. Obituary. *Br Med J* 1991;**302**:843.
8. Mitchell JRA. Diet and arterial disease — the myths and the realities. *Proc Nutr Soc* 1985;**44**:363–70.
9. Oliver M. Dietary cholesterol, plasma cholesterol and coronary heart disease. *Br Heart J* 1976;**38**:214–18.
10. Mitchell JR. What do we gain by modifying risk factors for coronary disease? *Schweiz Med Wochenschr* 1990;**120**:359–64.
11. Smith EB, Slater RS. Relationship between low-density lipoprotein in aortic intima and serum-lipid levels. *Lancet* 1972;**1**:463–9.
12. Slack J. Risks of ischaemic heart-disease in familial hyperlipoproteinaemic states. *Lancet* 1969;**2**:1380–2.
13. Soutar AK. Cholesterol, atherosclerosis and coronary disease in the UK, 1950–2000. In Reynolds LA, Tansey EM (eds.), *Wellcome Witnesses to Twentieth Century Medicine*, Vol. 21, 2006, p. 12.
14. French J. Atherosclerosis [Chapter 17]. In Florey H (ed.), *General Pathology* (2nd edn.). London: Lloyd-Luke (Medical Books) Ltd, 1958, pp. 351–377.
15. Sinclair HM. Deficiency of essential fatty acids and atherosclerosis, etcetera. *Lancet* 1956;**270**:381–3.

16. Sinclair HM. Prevention of coronary heart disease: The role of essential fatty acids. *Postgrad Med J* 1980;**56**:579–84.
17. Sinclair HM. The relative importance of essential fatty acids of the linoleic and linolenic families: Studies with an Eskimo diet. *Prog Lipid Res* 1981;**20**:897–9.

10 The Discovery of Statins

Canada

In 1981, I was fortunate to be the recipient of the Lucien Award for research into cardiovascular disease, awarded under the aegis of McGill University. A condition of the award was that I should spend 3 months working as a Visiting Professor with Allan Sniderman, a charismatic cardiologist with a major interest in lipids, at the Royal Victoria Hospital in Montreal. Allan had done his PhD with Dan Steinberg and my stay proved both scientifically profitable and socially enjoyable. Our research involved comparing the turnover of radiolabelled very low density lipoprotein (VLDL) and LDL in normal subjects, subjects with increased levels of apoB-containing lipoproteins in plasma, a condition with the catchy title hyperapobetalipoproteinaemia (hyperapoB), and patients with heterozygous FH. Analysis of the data showed that the increase in apoB in hyperapoB was solely due to increased synthesis of LDL secondary to increased synthesis of its precursor VLDL whereas in FH there was both increased synthesis of LDL, which was partly VLDL independent, as well as reduced LDL catabolism.[1] Hence, we showed that the two conditions exhibited distinctly different metabolic phenotypes.

My visit took place from December 1981 to February 1982 so I soon got to know the feel of a real Canadian winter. Jogging through the snow on Mont Royal was considerably more bracing than jogging along the bayous in the Houston heat (Figure 1). Also, the Lucien award was sufficiently rewarding financially for me to be able to take up skiing for the first time in my life, aged 49. On one occasion after a day's skiing at Mont Orford, a resort in the Eastern Townships, I went back to my car and started the

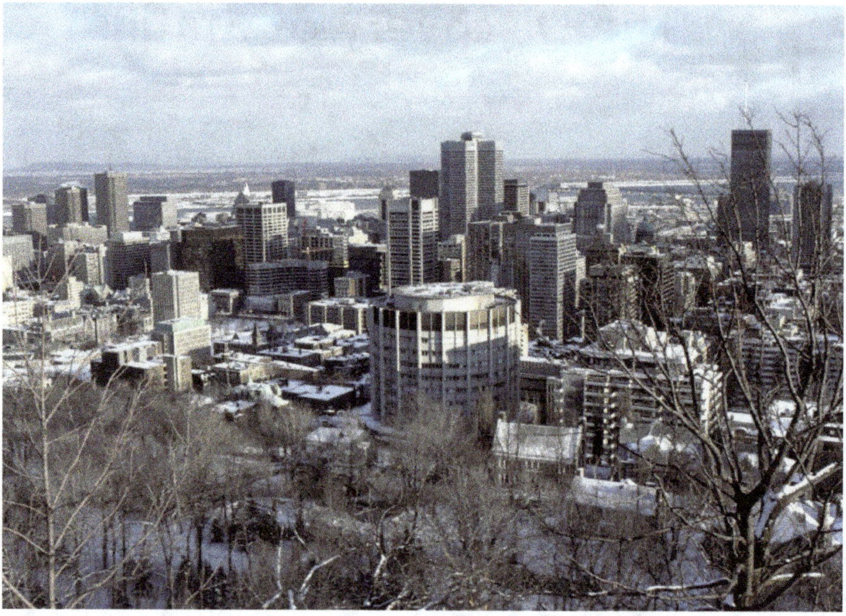

Figure 1. Downtown Montreal seen from Mont Royal with the St. Lawrence River in the background.

engine to warm the car up but inadvertently locked myself out. As the car got warmer I got colder and had it not been for a charitable French Canadian's expertise with a coat hanger, with which he managed to open the car door, I would have spent a very uncomfortable night in the car park, with the temperature already at −30°C and still falling.

While in Montreal, I paid a visit to the city of Quebec where the mid-winter Ice Carnival was in full swing. Some of the shops sold bottles of the local alcoholic "anti-freeze" called Caribou. Before buying this, customers first had to be scrutinised by the vendor to ensure they were over 18. Once this was established a label was stuck on one's jacket which stated "Il le capable d'en prendre" (he can take it)! Unfortunately, some took too much of it and fell asleep outside, running the risk of frostbite or even death during the bitterly cold nights.

About a year before I went to Canada, Neil McIntyre whom I knew in Boston, had referred one of his patients at the Royal Free Hospital for a trial of plasma exchange. She had primary biliary cirrhosis (a rare autoimmune liver disorder) which caused severe hypercholesterolaemia and xanthomatous neuropathy (nerve damage caused by the accumulation of cholesterol). The latter resulted in such intense hyperaesthesia (extreme sensitivity to touch) of her fingers that it was too painful for her to turn the key in the latch of her front door. Neil had previously introduced me to a friend of his, an expatriate clinical pharmacologist from the USA called Jonathan Tobert, who was visiting his family in London at the time. Jonathan worked for Merck at Rahway, New Jersey, and was involved in clinical trials of a new cholesterol synthesis inhibitor called mevinolin.[2] He kindly provided us with a small supply of this compound and we used it for 3 months on a compassionate use basis as an adjunct to plasma exchange. This combined therapy temporarily improved control of Neil's patient's hypercholesterolaemia and decreased the severity of her xanthomatous neuropathy. When her case was presented on the Staff Round we may have realised that this was the first time a statin had been used in Britain but we had no idea that this class of drug would eventually revolutionise the management of atherosclerotic cardiovascular disease throughout the world.

Akira Endo

The story of the discovery of statins starts in 1971 when Akira Endo, a Japanese microbiologist working for the pharmaceutical company Sankyo, began searching for microbial metabolites that would inhibit hydroxymethylglutaryl co-enzyme A reductase (HMG-CoA reductase), the key enzyme of cholesterol biosynthesis. His hopes that this would provide a novel means of lowering plasma cholesterol were vindicated when, after testing more than 6,000 microbial strains, he and his colleagues isolated a potent inhibitor of HMG CoA reductase from *Penicillium citrinum*, which lowered serum cholesterol in experimental animals.[3,4] Initially known as compactin, this compound was later called mevastatin and became the first HMG CoA reductase inhibitor, or statin, to be tested in humans.

Endo was born in November, 1933 in Akita Prefecture in the north east of Japan. His war time childhood was a rather sombre affair but was enlivened by his grandfather who used to take him mushroom picking in the nearby hills, engendering in him a lifelong interest in fungi. He excelled in Chemistry at high school and got a scholarship to Tohuku University, Sendai, where he studied Biotechnology. Immediately after graduating in 1957, he joined the Sankyo Company in Tokyo where his first project as a member of the applied microbiology group was to develop an enzyme that could be used to hydrolyse pectins contaminating wines and ciders. He successfully achieved this and was awarded his PhD by Tohoku University in 1966. For the next 2 years he did postdoctoral studies in the Department of Molecular Biology at the Albert Einstein College of Medicine in New York. After returning to Japan, he rejoined Sankyo and started his search for a microbial inhibitor of cholesterol biosynthesis.

Discovery of Compactin

Endo's premise that inhibition of HMG CoA reductase would lower plasma cholesterol was based on work conducted at the University of Texas in Dallas in the 1960s and was supported by Goldstein and Brown's discovery there in 1973 that FH is characterized by defective regulation of HMG CoA reductase. Using the cultured fibroblast system which they had devised, they and Endo showed compactin to be a potent inhibitor of cholesterol synthesis *in vitro* in cells from both normal subjects and patients with homozygous FH.[5,6] Initial *in vivo* studies in mice and rats were disappointingly negative,[7] but Endo persevered and showed that compactin lowered serum cholesterol in dogs and monkeys.[8,9] Interestingly, compactin had been isolated from a different mould by scientists at Beecham Laboratories in Britain at about the same time as Endo's discovery in Japan.[10] However, they did not investigate its effects on cholesterol synthesis until 1980 and lost interest in the compound when it failed to lower serum cholesterol in chicks and rats,[11] despite evidence that it inhibited cholesterol synthesis in human tissue.[12] Without doubt this was a missed opportunity.

The first clinical studies with compactin were carried out in Osaka by Yamamoto and Sudo in collaboration with Endo.[13] They showed that compactin in doses of 50–150 mg/day reduced serum cholesterol by 27% in patients with heterozygous FH, most of the decrease being in LDL cholesterol, but that higher doses were needed to lower cholesterol significantly in FH homozygotes. However, at that stage, Sankyo abruptly suspended their clinical trial programme, reputedly because of the perceived carcinogenicity of high doses of compactin in dogs. As a consequence, it was never licensed for use in man.

Endo left Sankyo in 1978 for an Associate Professorship in the School of Agriculture of Tokyo Noko University, where he continued his studies of fungal inhibitors of cholesterol synthesis. He had collaborated with the US drug company Merck several years previously by providing them with samples of compactin. The head of research at Merck at that time, Roy Vagelos, had a long-standing interest in HMG CoA reductase, and, like Endo he realized the therapeutic potential of inhibiting this enzyme. In 1980, his colleague Alberts and others at Merck discovered a second HMG CoA reductase inhibitor, which they isolated from *Aspergillus terreus*.[2] This was initially called mevinolin but was later renamed lovastatin. Endo isolated the same compound simultaneously but independently from a different mould, naming it "monocolin K."[14] He went on to discover several other HMG CoA reductase inhibitors over the next few years, became a full professor in 1986, and retired from the university in 1997. I got to know him quite well over the years during my many visits to Japan and I liked his quiet, dignified approach to life and his understated sense of humour.

Lovastatin

Merck proceeded with the clinical development of lovastatin, but the suspension of all clinical studies with compactin by Sankyo put them in a quandary, especially since Sankyo would not disclose the reason. After much deliberation, Merck followed suit and stopped all clinical work while they undertook additional safety studies in animals. The results were sufficiently reassuring for them to resume clinical trials with lovastatin in 1983 and 4 years later it became the first HMG CoA reductase inhibitor to be licensed by the US Food and Drug Administration (FDA).[15] In the interim, Tobert arranged for the compound to be made available to treat patients with refractory FH on a named patient basis, and I and my Hammersmith colleagues gratefully took advantage of this facility from 1983 onwards, with encouraging results.

The ability to treat these severely hypercholesterolaemic patients effectively and safely with such a well-tolerated compound represented a major therapeutic advance, especially since its LDL-lowering effect of over 30% was additive to that of existing therapies such as cholestyramine, partial ileal bypass and apheresis. We published our observations, the first description of the clinical use of a statin in Britain, in the *Quarterly Journal of Medicine* (*QJM*) in 1986.[16] Using radiolabelled LDL, we and also others showed that by inhibiting HMG CoA reductase, lovastatin stimulated receptor-mediated LDL uptake *in vivo*, thereby compensating for the partial deficiency of LDL receptors in FH heterozygotes. However, like Yamamoto, we found that FH homozygotes were less responsive than heterozygotes, a reflection of their near total lack of LDL receptors. Because of patent constraints exerted by Sankyo lovastatin was never licensed in Britain, but Merck maintained supplies for compassionate use until 1989, when its successor simvastatin was licensed here. As will become clear later, the latter compound played a key role in vindicating the lipid hypothesis.

Other Statins

Other statins soon followed, including pravastatin in 1991, which was derived from compactin and developed by Sankyo; fluvastatin in 1994, which was the first synthetic HMG CoA reductase inhibitor; atorvastatin and cerivastatin in 1997; and rosuvastatin in 2003, the latest and most potent of these compounds to be licensed in the UK and capable of reducing LDL by over 50%. Myotoxicity (muscle damage) leading to rhabdomyolysis (breakdown and release of muscle protein into the circulation) is the only serious side effect of statins, but is rare with an incidence of under 0.1%. It is reversible when the statin is stopped, but if not diagnosed, it can lead to renal failure and sometimes death.

The discovery of statins by Endo resulted in huge profits for the pharmaceutical industry, but it was not all plain sailing. In addition to early concerns over the suspected toxicity of compactin, atorvastatin was nearly scrapped by Parke-Davis on economic grounds. It is said that Roger Newton, who was deeply involved in its development, literally went down on his knees before the board of directors to plead for its continuation. The directors relented and it later became the best-selling drug in the world. In contrast, cerivastatin was withdrawn by its manufacturer Bayer in 2001 after 31 deaths from rhabdomyolysis had been reported, an outcome that cost Bayer $600 million in out of court settlements in the USA.

Compassionate Use of Lovastatin in the UK

Much of the success of the clinical development and marketing of lovastatin by Merck was due to the clinical trial data meticulously gathered by Jonathan Tobert. In Britain, it was available on a compassionate use basis only in a limited number of centres, one of which was the Hammersmith. Consequently, the Lipid Clinic there had numerous referrals from other parts of the country of hypercholesterolaemic patients who were refractory to conventional drug therapy.

My colleagues and I now began treating a small number of FH patients with lipoprotein apheresis combined with lovastatin, which radically reduced their LDL cholesterol levels. Using computer-assisted quantitative angiography, now performed by cardiologists working with radiologists, it was possible to show quite marked regression of coronary lesions in some of these patients after 1–2 years of apheresis and lovastatin (Figure 2). Although our results were anecdotal and by no means constituted scientific proof, the angiographic images were evocative[17] and I received numerous invitations to speak at meetings all over the world. Many of these meetings

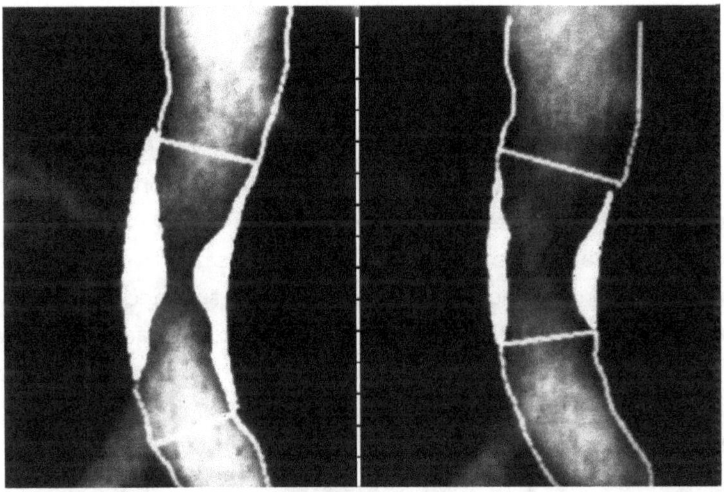

Figure 2. Computer-assisted angiograms of the coronary artery of a hypercholesterolaemic patient before (left) and after (right) 18 months treatment with lipoprotein apheresis and lovastatin, showing regression of an atheromatous plaque (reproduced with permission from Ref. 17).

were sponsored by drug companies, which in those days were far more generous in their financial support for such events than is permitted nowadays. As a result, I travelled to some exotic places and stayed in some very grand hotels, including the Al Mamounia in Marrakech and the Negresco in Nice. Another memorable experience was staying in a ryokan, a traditional Japanese hotel, in Kanazawa and visiting the local geisha house.

Travel to these meetings could sometimes be somewhat fraught, such as when I took an Aeroflot flight from Moscow to Sochi on the Black Sea. One of my fellow passengers, a Finn, was so unnerved by the near vertical take-off of our Ilyushin airliner and the accompanying sounds of breaking crockery that he consumed an entire bottle of vodka during the 3-hour flight. After the plane had made its equally abrupt and noisy touch down (the captain must have been an ex-fighter pilot) the Finn stood up and letting out a cry of relief, swung the empty bottle around his head and collapsed in the aisle. He was carried off the plane by a couple of hefty Russian air hostesses and dumped on the tarmac. On another occasion I flew to Peshawar, Pakistan, in an ancient Boeing 707 which was packed full of bearded Afghan Mujahadeen, returning to their refugee camps after a shopping trip to Karachi. I was the only European on the plane and felt decidedly isolated. On arrival at my hotel in Peshawar I had to sign a statement that I was an alcoholic before I could buy a beer. At times I flew too frequently for my liking but not as frequently as some of my colleagues; one of them, a well-known Oxford cardiologist, found after he returned from one of his frequent trips abroad that some humourist had put a "Visitor to Britain" sticker on his car. However, flying to New York in Concorde to hear the results of the Helsinki Heart Study and British Airways first class to Tokyo to give a lecture are nostalgic memories of a bygone era.

Almost a century and a half ago, Mark Twain summed up the essence of research in these words: "Discovery! To know that you are walking where none others have walked; that you are beholding what human eye has not seen before … to discover a great thought, an intellectual nugget, right under the dust of a field that many a brain-plough has gone over before … To be the first — that is the idea."[18] Akira Endo's discovery of the hypocholesterolaemic properties of *Penicillium citrinum* was undoubtedly a first in the prevention and cure of atherosclerotic cardiovascular

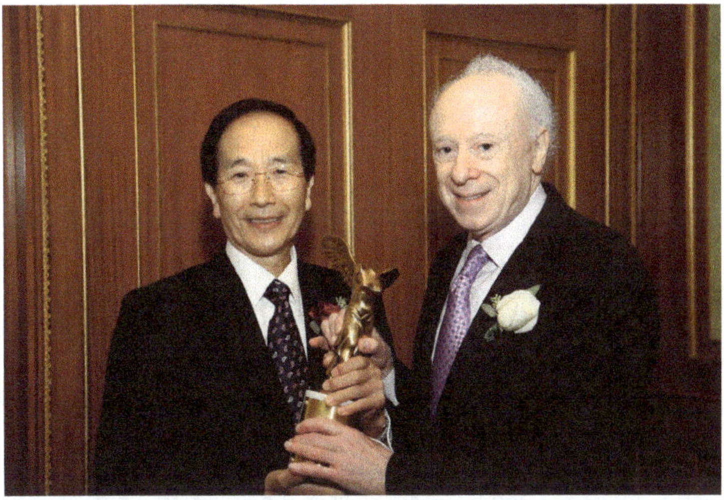

Figure 3. Akira Endo receiving the Lasker-DeBakey Clinical Research Award from Joe Goldstein in 2008 (reproduced from Ref. 19).

disease, just as Alexander Fleming's discovery half a century earlier of the antibiotic properties of *Penicillium notatum* revolutionized the treatment of bacterial infections. Many consider that Endo is just as deserving of the Nobel Prize as was Fleming, but, unlike the latter, he has not received it. Fittingly, however, he was given the Lasker Award for Clinical Research in 2008 (Figure 3) and the Gairdner International Award in 2017, these being generally regarded as the US and Canadian equivalents, respectively, of the Nobel Prize. I was proud to be among those who nominated him for both these awards.

References

1. Teng B, Sniderman AD, Soutar AK, Thompson GR. Metabolic basis of hyperapobetalipoproteinemia. Turnover of apolipoprotein B in low density lipoprotein and its precursors and subfractions compared with normal and familial hypercholesterolemia. *J Clin Invest* 1986;**77**:663–72.
2. Alberts AW, Chen J, Kuron G *et al.* Mevinolin: A highly potent competitive inhibitor of hydroxymethylglutaryl-coenzyme A reductase and a cholesterol-lowering agent. *Proc Natl Acad Sci USA* 1980;**77**:3957–61.

3. Endo A, Kuroda M, Tsujita Y. ML-236A, ML-236B, and ML-236C, new inhibitors of cholesterogenesis produced by *Penicillium citrinum*. *J Antibiot* 1976; **29**:1346–8.
4. Endo A, Kuroda M, Tanzawa K. Competitive inhibition of 3-hydroxy-3-methylglutaryl coenzyme A reductase by ML-236A and ML-236B fungal metabolites, having hypocholesterolemic activity. *FEBS Lett* 1976;**72**:323–6.
5. Kaneko I, Hazama-Shimada Y, Endo A. Inhibitory effects on lipid metabolism in cultured cells of ML-236B, a potent inhibitor of 3-hydroxy-3-methylgutaryl-coenzyme-A reductase. *Eur J Biochem* 1978;**87**:313–21.
6. Brown MS, Faust JR, Goldstein JL, Kaneko I, Endo A. Induction of 3-hydroxy-3-methylglutaryl coenzyme A reductase activity in human fibroblasts incubated with compactin (ML-236B), a competitive inhibitor of the reductase. *J Biol Chem* 1978;**253**:1121–8.
7. Endo A, Tsujita Y, Kuroda M, Tanzawa K. Effects of ML-236B on cholesterol metabolism in mice and rats: Lack of hypocholesterolemic activity in normal animals. *Biochim Biophys Acta* 1979;**575**:266–76.
8. Tsujita Y, Kuroda M, Tanzawa K, Kitano N, Endo A. Hypolipidemic effects in dogs of ML-236B, a competitive inhibitor of 3-hydroxy-3-methylglutaryl coenzyme A reductase. *Atherosclerosis* 1979;**32**:307–13.
9. Kuroda M, Tsujita Y, Tanzawa K, Endo A. Hypolipidemic effects in monkeys of ML-236B, a competitive inhibitor of 3-hydroxy-3-methylglutaryl coenzyme A reductase. *Lipids* 1979;**14**:585–9.
10. Steinberg D. An interpretative history of the cholesterol controversy. V. The discovery of the statins and the end of the controversy. *J Lipid Res* 2006;**47**:1339–51.
11. Fears R, Richards DH, Ferres H. The effect of compactin, a potent inhibitor of 3-hydroxy-3- methylglutaryl coenzyme-A reductase activity, on cholesterogenesis and serum cholesterol levels in rats and chicks. *Atherosclerosis* 1980;**35**:439–49.
12. Betteridge DJ, Krone W, Reckless JPD, Galton DJ. Compactin inhibits cholesterol synthesis in lymphocytes and intestinal mucosa from patients with familial hypercholesterolaemia. *Lancet* 1978;**2**:1342–3.
13. Yamamoto A, Sudo H, Endo A. Therapeutic effects of ML-236B in primary hypercholesterolemia. *Atherosclerosis* 1980;**35**:259–66.
14. Endo A. Monacolin K. A new hypocholesterolemic agent produced by a *Monascus* species. *J Antibiot* 1979;**32**:852–4.
15. Tobert JA. Lovastatin and beyond: The history of the HMG-CoA reductase inhibitors. *Nat Rev Drug Discov* 2003;**2**:517–26.

16. Thompson GR, Ford J, Jenkinson M, Trayner I. Efficacy of mevinolin as adjuvant therapy for refractory familial hypercholesterolaemia. *Q J Med* 1986;**60**:803–11.
17. Barbir M, Michishita I, Larkin S, Thompson GR. Computer analysed angiogram of a plaque in the circumflex artery of an hypercholesterolaemic patient before and after I8 months' treatment. *Br Med J* 1989;**298**:I32.
18. Twain, M. *The Innocents Abroad*. London: John Camden Hotten, 1869.
19. Thompson G, Mabuchi H. Akira Endo: The discovery of statins. In Thompson G (ed.), *Pioneers of Medicine without a Nobel Prize*. London: Imperial College Press, 2014, pp. 251–69.

11 Does Lowering Cholesterol Cause Murder and Suicide?

Cholesterol-Lowering in Coronary Prevention

The contrast between the persistently high death rate from coronary heart disease in England and Wales during the 1970s and rapidly falling rates in the USA and Australia led epidemiologists such as Geoffrey Rose to advocate the mass strategy or population approach to coronary prevention in Britain. This was based on the premise that in overall terms many more deaths occur in the large proportion of the population at low risk than in the much smaller proportion at high risk.[1] In contrast, Oliver, a clinician, supported the high-risk strategy, taking the view that the negative outcome of multifactorial risk factor intervention trials meant that the population approach would not work in practice, and discounting claims that the reduction in coronary mortality in the USA might have been due to lifestyle changes.[2] This view was reflected in 1987 by the recommendations of the British Cardiac Society Working Group on Coronary Prevention, of which he was the convener,[3] whereas the European Atherosclerosis Society and the British Hyperlipidaemia Association both hedged their bets and supported a combined high-risk and population approach.[4,5]

Two years earlier, the NIH had held a Consensus Conference on Lowering Blood Cholesterol to Prevent Heart Disease, under the chairmanship of Dan Steinberg.[6] This concluded that elevated blood cholesterol levels are a major cause of coronary disease and that lowering them would reduce the risk of heart attacks. It went on to recommend cholesterol screening and the treatment with diet or drugs of those found to have a

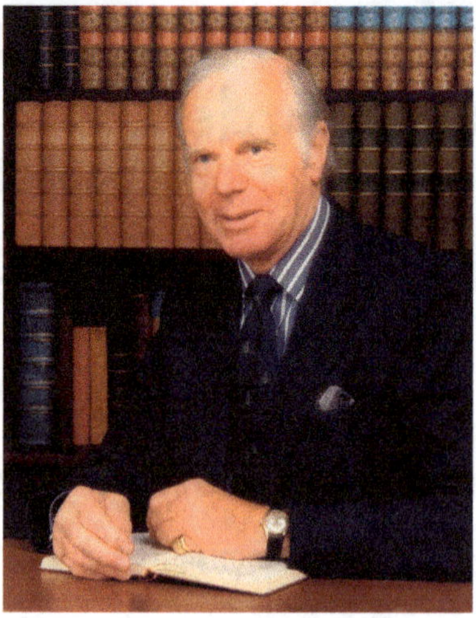

Figure 1. Michael Oliver (1925–2015).

raised value, as well as the adoption of dietary measures aimed at lowering the cholesterol level of the entire US population.

The findings of the Consensus Conference were criticised by Oliver[7] on the grounds that the outcome had been predetermined by the choice of experts invited to participate, although the various alternatives he proposed all seemed liable to the same source of bias (Figure 1). He later switched his line of attack on American efforts to prevent coronary heart disease by invoking safety concerns, pointing out that while lowering serum cholesterol reduced coronary mortality it failed to decrease total mortality, perhaps by increasing non-cardiovascular causes of death.[8] He went on to suggest that the presence of low cholesterol in patients with cancer was not necessarily a post-hoc phenomenon and that therapeutic lowering of serum cholesterol might sometimes cause cancer, possibly by altering the cholesterol content of cell membranes. The concept that lowering serum cholesterol might be carcinogenic was not new but dated from the Los Angeles Veterans Administration Trial conducted 20 years previously, where an increased risk of developing cancer was observed in men having a diet high in polyunsaturated fat. It so happened that the expression of these safety concerns was the prelude to a major escalation in hostilities on the cholesterol front.

Low Cholesterol and Violent Deaths

In 1990, Muldoon and two of his colleagues at the University of Pittsburgh, a psychologist and a psychiatrist, published in the *British Medical Journal BMJ*) a meta-analysis of six primary prevention trials of cholesterol reduction, two using diet, and four using drugs.[9] Coronary mortality was shown to be significantly reduced by drug treatment, but total mortality was unchanged. This reflected a significant increase in deaths from accidents, suicide and violence in those on treatment, although there was no correlation between cholesterol reduction and deaths from cancer. The authors were unable to provide a plausible explanation as to why lowering serum cholesterol should predispose to violent deaths, but they considered the possibility that it did so by altering neuronal function. They subsequently suggested that cholesterol-lowering manoeuvres might reduce brain serotoninergic activity (serotonin is a neurotransmitter that is thought to exert a beneficial influence on mood) and thereby promote aggressive tendencies and suicidal behaviour.[10]

One of the studies analysed in Muldoon's original meta-analysis was the Minnesota Coronary Survey, during which inmates of six mental hospitals who had been on a lipid-lowering diet for just over a year had a significant excess of accidental deaths when compared with inmates not on the diet. The causes of death included fractures, drug reactions, burns, foreign bodies, tooth extractions, freezing, heatstroke, drowning and suicide. It is hard to conceive of a unifying causal mechanism which could account for such a wide and disparate range of fatal events.[11]

Evidence from other sources did not support the findings of Muldoon *et al.* In the Whitehall Study, almost 18,000 men were followed up for 20 years, during which 90 died from accidents, violence or suicide. No significant association was seen between these deaths and serum cholesterol at entry to the study.[12] A large Swedish study did find a negative correlation between serum cholesterol at entry and suicide within the next 7 years, but not during the remainder of the 20 years of follow-up, and the increased risk of suicide was seen only in men, not in women.[13] A similar study in Finland showed no association between serum cholesterol and violent deaths or suicides during 10–15 years of follow-up but found these deaths to be more prevalent among smokers and drinkers.[14] These findings may have reassured some, but not Michael Oliver, who continued to sound the alarm in editorials with titles such as *Might treatment of hypercholesterolaemia increase non-cardiac mortality?* and *Is cholesterol reduction always safe?*

Supposed Dangers of Cholesterol-Lowering Drugs

Anxieties over this issue were suddenly brought to public attention in 1992 with the publication of an article by George Davey Smith and Juha Pekkanen titled *Should there be a moratorium on the use of cholesterol lowering drugs?*[15] This was at a time when the development of statins was proceeding at a rapid pace and clinical trials with lovastatin, simvastatin and pravastatin were underway. Davey Smith and Pekkanen had conducted a meta-analysis similar to but larger than Muldoon's, including additional data from diet and drug trials. They confirmed that coronary mortality was reduced by lowering cholesterol in both types of trial and that total mortality was unchanged. However, they also reported a highly significant increase in non-coronary mortality, reflecting an amalgam of cancer, injury and other non-cardiovascular causes of death in the intervention groups of the drug trials, but not the diet trials. This led them to question whether the general use of cholesterol-lowering drugs was justified and to propose that the prescription of these agents should be restricted to patients with familial hyperlipidaemia until the results of the statin trials became known, still some years hence.

The publication of this paper in the *BMJ* resulted in an immediate plethora of hyperbolical headlines in the newspapers, ranging from "Heart pills may kill you" to "Murders linked to low-fat drugs", causing panic among patients who were on cholesterol-lowering medication and disquiet to their doctors (Figure 2). Public and professional anxiety regarding the safety of these compounds persisted until 1994, when Malcolm Law and his colleagues conducted an exhaustively thorough, systematic review of 40 published studies.[16] Apart from an unexplained increase in the risk of fatal haemorrhagic stroke in hypertensive subjects, they found no evidence that lowering or having a low cholesterol increased mortality from any cause. They attributed the associations between low serum cholesterol and both

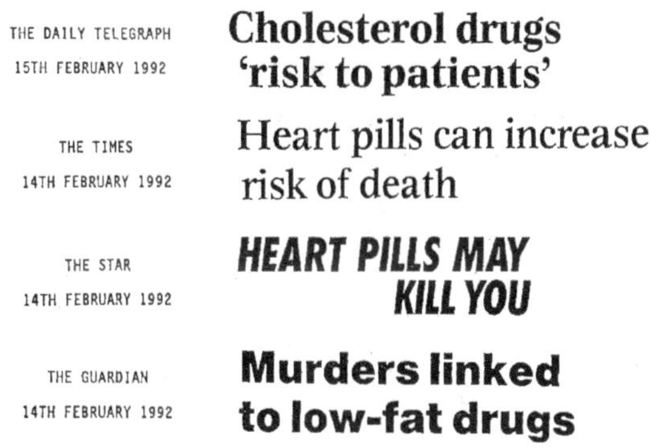

THE DAILY TELEGRAPH
15TH FEBRUARY 1992
Cholesterol drugs 'risk to patients'

THE TIMES
14TH FEBRUARY 1992
Heart pills can increase risk of death

THE STAR
14TH FEBRUARY 1992
HEART PILLS MAY KILL YOU

THE GUARDIAN
14TH FEBRUARY 1992
Murders linked to low-fat drugs

Figure 2. Newspaper headlines proclaiming the purported risks of cholesterol-lowering drugs.

cancer and suicide to confounding, in as much as low serum cholesterol is often a consequence of cancer or of dietary neglect, the latter being a common finding in depressed subjects with suicidal tendencies. An accompanying editorial in the *BMJ* damned their conclusions with faint praise with its subtitle: *Lowering population cholesterol concentrations probably isn't harmful.*

For conveying the impression that the excess mortality in a number of the drug trials was spurious, Law *et al*, were criticised by Oliver and his colleagues, who emphasised that the increased mortality of subjects on clofibrate in the WHO trial was genuine,[17] whereas Davey Smith and Egger took the issue with them on their use of statistics.[18] Muldoon, too, was initially reluctant to accept that cholesterol-lowering measures were safe, but he and his colleagues later acknowledged that "currently available evidence does not indicate that non-cholesterol illness mortality is increased significantly by cholesterol lowering treatments."[19] Despite the criticisms, Law's analysis did a great deal to reassure those responsible for prescribing lipid-lowering drugs at a time when the latter were under intense scrutiny and the safety of statins was still an unknown quantity.

Pseudo-Scientific Gobbledegook

Public unease about cholesterol continued, however, fuelled by individuals within the medical profession and news media alike. This was exemplified by an article in the *Sunday Express* in 1990 with the pejorative title *Exploding the cholesterol myth.*[20] The medical editor who wrote the article suggested that "raised cholesterol might be a symptom, rather than a cause, of a state in which heart disease became likely ... Raised levels of circulating cholesterol should be seen as a reflection of the over-taxed body's attempts to cope with these demands." The article went on to point out that lowering cholesterol might be harmful and concluded, "because of the hazards of long-term treatment, the wise patient will make every effort to come off the drugs as soon as possible." The likely source of this pseudoscientific nonsense is revealed in the following excerpts from a letter written that year by a consultant cardiologist at a London teaching hospital to one of his patients:

> Dear Mr C
> This is just a letter to confirm my opinion that you live with high levels of adrenergic drive by habit, sufficiently high as to carry you over the top of the curve into catabolic territory where the cholesterol level naturally climbs...
>
> If you learned to live at the peak instead of on the downslope of the curve I would expect your cholesterol levels to regress from their excursions towards a mean. As far as I know, this mean may be within the normal range of values.

It seems likely that the journalist picked up the notion that a raised cholesterol is a post-hoc phenomenon from the cardiologist who wrote that bizarre letter. Unfortunately, some believed what they read in the newspaper, including a patient who had undergone coronary bypass surgery and whose hypercholesterolaemia was being treated at a Northampton hospital. The consultant in charge wrote to the paper's editor, complaining that his patient had discontinued all cholesterol-lowering medication after reading the article in question and was now untreated. The likelihood is that he and other patients who reacted in a similar manner sustained potentially serious consequences. These anecdotes illustrate that the cholesterol controversy was by no means dead and buried at the start of the statin era and that it continued to influence the actions of doctors and patients alike.

References

1. Rose G. Strategy of prevention: Lessons from cardiovascular disease. *Br Med J* 1981;**282**:1847–51.
2. Oliver MF. Should we not forget about mass control of coronary risk factors? *Lancet* 1983;**2**:37–38.
3. British Cardiac Society Working Group on Coronary Prevention. Conclusions and recommendations. *Br Heart J* 1987;**57**:188–9.
4. Study Group, European Atherosclerosis Society. Strategies for the prevention of coronary heart disease: A policy statement of the European Atherosclerosis Society. *Eur Heart J* 1987;**8**:77–88.
5. Shepherd J, Betteridge DJ, Durrington P *et al.* Strategies for reducing coronary heart disease and desirable limits for blood lipid concentrations: Guidelines of the British Hyperlipidaemia Association. *Br Med J* 1987;**295**:1245–6.
6. Consensus Conference. Lowering blood cholesterol to prevent heart disease. *JAMA* 1985;**253**:2080–6.
7. Oliver MF. Consensus or nonsensus — Conferences on coronary heart disease. *Lancet* 1985;**1**:1087–9.
8. Oliver MF. Reducing cholesterol does not reduce mortality. *J Am Coll Cardiol* 1988;**12**:814–17.
9. Muldoon MF, Manuck SB, Matthews KA. Lowering cholesterol concentrations and mortality: A quantitative review of primary prevention trials. *Br Med J* 1990;**301**:309–14.
10. Muldoon MF, Rossouw JE, Manuck CB, Glueck CJ, Kaplan JR, Kaufmann PG. Low or lowered cholesterol and risk of death from suicide and trauma. *Metabolism* 1993;**42**(Suppl 1):45–56.
11. Thompson GR. Cholesterol lowering and non-cardiac mortality [Letter]. *Lancet* 1991;**2**:126.
12. Davey Smith G, Shipley MJ, Marmot MG, Patel C. Lowering cholesterol concentrations and mortality [Letter]. *Br Med J* 1990;**301**:552.
13. Lindberg G, Rastam L, Gullberg B, Eklund GA. Low serum cholesterol concentrations and short term mortality from injuries in men and women. *Br Med J* 1992;**305**:277–9.
14. Vartiainen E, Puska P, Pekkanen J, Tuomilehto J, Lönnqvist J, Ehnholm C. Serum cholesterol concentration and mortality from accidents, suicide, and other violent causes. *Br Med J* 1994;**309**:445–7.
15. Davey Smith G, Pekkanen J. Should there be a moratorium on the use of cholesterol lowering drugs? *Br Med J* 1992;**304**:431–4.

16. Law MR, Thompson SG, Wald NJ. Assessing possible hazards of reducing serum cholesterol. *Br Med J* 1994;**308**:373–9.
17. Heady JA, Morris JN, Oliver MF. Ischaemic heart disease and cholesterol… and mislead on adverse effects [Letter]. *Br Med J* 1994;**308**:1040.
18. Smith GD, Egger M. Commentary: Statistical problems. *Br Med J* 1994;**308**:1025–7.
19. Muldoon MF, Manuck SB, Mendelsohn AB, Kaplan JR, Belle SH. Cholesterol reduction and non-illness mortality: Meta-analysis of randomised clinical trials. *Br Med J* 2001;**322**:11–15.
20. Hodgkinson N. Exploding the cholesterol myth. *Sunday Express*, 4 February 1990.

12 The Statin Trials Prove the Lipid Hypothesis

Testing the Lipid Hypothesis

Despite the efforts of epidemiologists, lipidologists, and others, many cardiologists remained unconvinced that lowering cholesterol by diet or drugs would provide an effective, let alone safe, means of treating and preventing coronary heart disease. However, there were some who accepted that cholesterol might play a causal role in atherosclerosis and they set out to test this hypothesis by undertaking so-called regression trials, in which the impact of cholesterol-lowering measures on hyperlipidaemic patients with coronary artery disease was assessed angiographically by injecting radio-opaque dye during cardiac catheterisation and obtaining X-ray cine images of their coronary arteries before and after treatment.

Angiographic Regression Trials

The results of a dozen such studies between 1984 and 1994 were summarised in an editorial by the author.[1] Most of these were from the USA and they ranged in size from less than 50 to over 800 subjects and lasted between 1 and 10 years. The majority involved a randomized comparison of the effects of diet versus diet combined with lipid-lowering drugs. Alternative forms of treatment included partial ileal bypass, exercise, and anti-stress measures. In the earlier trials, drugs that prevented reabsorption of bile acids, such as cholestyramine and colestipol, were given alone or in combination with either nicotinic acid or lovastatin. In the later trials, lovastatin or simvastatin were given as monotherapy. Likewise in the earlier trials, angiographic changes were assessed visually by radiologists, whereas the later trials employed computer-assisted quantitative coronary angiography (QCA). The latter method was used in the MAAS trial in which Hammersmith Hospital was one of the participating centres, the others being in Holland, Sweden, Germany, Belgium, and France. I was a member of the Steering Committee of MAAS which was chaired by Michael Oliver, whom I got to know well and to like, despite our views on lipids diverging at times.

Baseline levels of serum total and LDL cholesterol varied considerably between the 12 trials, with overall means of 6.3 and 4.4 mmol/L, respectively (values regarded as normal at that time would have been less than 5 and 3 mmol/L, respectively). During the trials, LDL cholesterol was 31% lower in the intervention groups than in the controls. Angiographic criteria varied between trials but all patients were categorized according to whether their coronary atherosclerotic lesions showed progression, regression, mixed response, or no change. Of the more than 2,500 patients involved, 44% of the controls were classified as progressors and 9% as regressors, compared with 29% and 18%, respectively, of those on drug treatment. Hence, effective LDL-lowering treatment reduced the likelihood of progression by one-third and increased the chances of regression two-fold.

Although not designed to detect changes in clinical end points, some trials did show a significant reduction in cardiovascular events and in the need for revascularization procedures such as coronary artery bypass grafting.[2–4] Greg Brown *et al.* in Seattle examined the relation between clinical events and atherosclerotic plaque size in one of these trials,[3] and concluded that mild to moderately stenosed coronary lesions were usually the culprits of clinical events and were more responsive to lipid-lowering therapy than were more severely stenosed lesions.[5]

As was shown by the late Michael Davies (who was a keen flyfisherman) and his colleagues at St. George's in London, high-grade stenotic lesions contain large amounts of collagen and calcium but relatively little lipid, whereas the propensity of plaques to undergo fissuring and thrombosis, and thereby precipitate a clinical event such as a heart attack, was determined by the amount of cholesterol in the core of the plaque.[6] Thus, a reduction in the amount of lipid in moderately stenotic lesions resulting in only a modest decrease in plaque size should be accompanied by an increase in plaque stability and fewer clinical events, as indeed was observed in the Seattle trial.

In September 1992, a joint meeting of the British Atherosclerosis Discussion Group and the European Atherosclerosis Society was held at Downing College in Cambridge, organised by Alan Howard and myself. The topic was "Regression of atherosclerosis" and the participants included several of those who had made major contributions in this field, notably Michael Davies, Greg Brown, and David Blankenhorn. The careful pathological studies of Davies and Woolf were hailed as being especially important in showing that lesion composition, rather than plaque stenotic severity, was the main factor in determining clinical events. All participants agreed that the regression trials provided a strong hint that lipid-lowering therapy could reduce coronary events, but the question of whether or not this would be accompanied by a reduction in total mortality, the Holy Grail of cardiologists, was still unresolved. The answer was not long in coming, however, and it came from Scandinavia.

4S

In the autumn of 1994, *The Lancet* published the results of the Scandinavian Simvastatin Survival Study (4S), which provided unequivocal evidence that treatment of hypercholesterolaemia in patients with pre-existing coronary heart disease reduced both cardiovascular events and total mortality.[7] In this epic trial, 4,444 mostly male patients from Denmark, Finland, Iceland, Norway, and Sweden, aged 35–70 with angina or previous myocardial infarction (heart attack) and with serum cholesterol averaging 6.8 mmol/L while on diet, were randomized to receive simvastatin or placebo. Simvastatin dosage was initially 20 mg/day but was increased to 40 mg/day as necessary, so as to maintain serum cholesterol in the range 3–5.2 mmol/L. During the study, simvastatin reduced total cholesterol by 25% and LDL cholesterol by 35%.

The median duration of treatment was 5.4 years, after which the trial was stopped because of a highly significant 30% reduction in total mortality. This was entirely due to a 42% reduction in coronary mortality, and there was no increase in non-cardiovascular causes of death, including cancer and trauma. In addition to its effects on coronary disease, simvastatin significantly reduced the occurrence of strokes. The mean level of LDL cholesterol with simvastatin in 4S was 3.2 mmol/L, similar to the 3 mmol/L seen in the regression trials. Taken together with the latter, these findings showed that a 30–35% reduction in LDL cholesterol resulted in decreased progression and increased regression of coronary atheromatous lesions and fewer cardiovascular events; the 4S authors estimated that simvastatin had prevented 4 out of every 9 deaths that otherwise would have occurred.

The publication of the 4S results had an immediate impact on medical practice. Even Michael Oliver was impressed, and he was co-author of an article in the *BMJ* titled "Lower patients' cholesterol now."[8] However, this included a caveat that the increase in non-cardiovascular mortality seen in some primary prevention trials of cholesterol lowering was still an issue to be resolved.

WHO Trial of Clofibrate

Oliver's reservations concerning safety arose from the WHO double-blind, multicentre trial of primary prevention in over 15,000 men aged 30–59, which he had initiated in 1965.[9] All participants were free from coronary heart disease at the start and were observed for just over 5 years. The treatment group, consisting of more than 5,000 men whose serum cholesterol averaged 6.8 mmol/l, received the lipid-lowering drug clofibrate 1.6 g/day, and a matching control group received a placebo. Serum cholesterol decreased by 9% in the clofibrate group, and this was associated with a 25% decrease in non-fatal myocardial infarcts compared with the control group. However, the incidence of fatal myocardial infarcts in the two groups was similar, and the crude death rate was actually higher in clofibrate-treated subjects, mainly due to an excess of deaths from diseases involving the liver, most notably gallstones. The results suggested that lowering the serum cholesterol level reduced the incidence of coronary heart disease, but that clofibrate had too many disadvantages to be used for this purpose in the general population.

The latter impression was reinforced 2 years later when the WHO investigators published an analysis of over 5 years of in-trial and more than 4 years of follow-up data.[10] This showed that clofibrate-treated subjects had sustained a 25% increase in total mortality, which sounded the death knell for the drug. It also posed difficult questions for adherents of the lipid hypothesis and undoubtedly raised serious doubts in Michael Oliver's mind about the safety of cholesterol-lowering therapy in general, doubts which influenced his attitude to coronary prevention for many years afterwards.

WOSCOPS

An answer to this safety issue would soon be forthcoming from the West of Scotland Coronary Primary Prevention Study (WOSCOPS).[11] The latter was conceived by Jim Shepherd at the Glasgow Royal Infirmary in 1988 during a visit there by a senior director of Squibb, the licensee in Britain of pravastatin.[12] Shepherd suggested that a primary prevention trial (i.e. conducted in patients without coronary disease) was needed, an idea which appealed to Squibb. As a result WOSCOPS became the first primary prevention trial to use a statin. This initially involved screening more than 80,000 men in the West of Scotland, of whom 6,595 were selected on the basis of being asymptomatic, aged 45–64 and having serum total cholesterol over 6.5 mmol/L and LDL cholesterol of 4.5–6 mmol/L. They were then randomized to receive pravastatin 40 mg/day or placebo for an average duration of just under 5 years.

The results were published in 1995, exactly a year after the publication of 4S. Pravastatin decreased serum total and LDL cholesterol by 20% and 26%, respectively, these changes being associated with a highly significant 31% reduction in non-fatal myocardial infarcts plus coronary deaths. Although the 22% reduction in total mortality just failed to achieve statistical significance, there was no increase in non-cardiovascular causes of death in pravastatin-treated subjects. This suggested that the contrary findings of the WHO trial reflected the mechanism of action of clofibrate, which promotes gallstone formation, not the effect of cholesterol-lowering *per se*.

The British Hyperlipidaemia Association and HEART UK

The origins of the British Hyperlipidaemia Association and HEART UK date back to 1985 when Jim Shepherd, who was subsequently the lead investigator of WOSCOPS, convened a meeting of the "Lipid Clinics Group" at Hammersmith Hospital. The inaugural scientific meeting of the British Association of Lipid Disorders (BALD) took place the following year and he was elected Chairman (Figure 1). It was renamed the British Hyperlipidaemia Association (BHA) in 1987 and, in 2003, HEART UK. The Myant Lecture, commemorating Nick Myant's contribution to lipid research in the UK, was

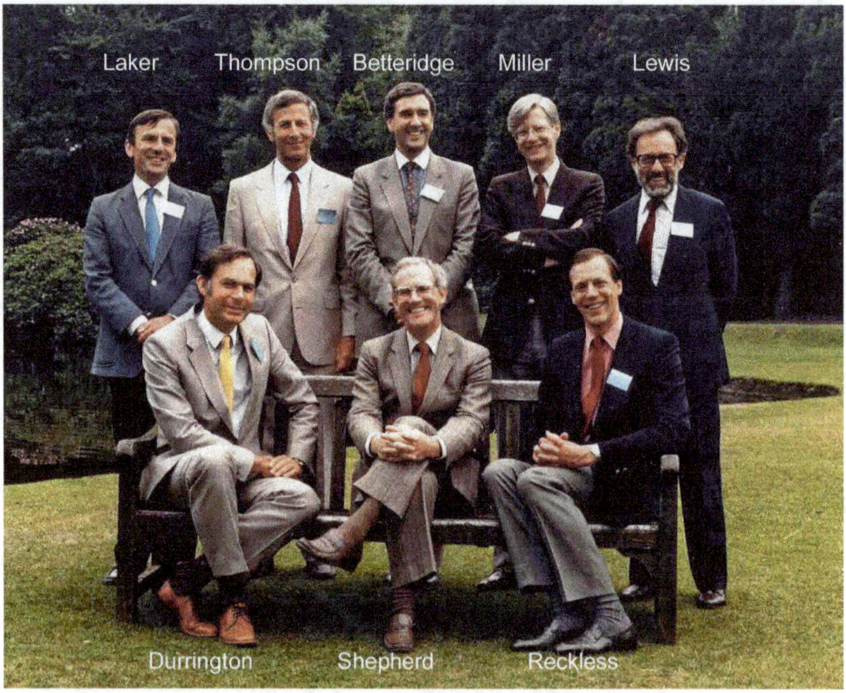

Figure 1. Committee of the British Association for Lipid Disorders in 1986, precursor of the British Hyperlipidaemia Association and HEART UK.

inaugurated in 1989 and has been given at the annual meetings of the society by a number of distinguished speakers including, after I succeeded Jim Shepherd as BHA Chairman, Joe Goldstein.

Over the past 30 years, the BHA/HEART UK has been actively involved in advancing lipid-lowering therapy in the UK. BHA guidelines on lipid-lowering to prevent coronary heart disease (CHD) were published in 1987 and 1993 and the BHA was a signatory to the Joint British Guidelines on prevention of CHD in 1998 and, as HEART UK, in 2005. HEART UK working groups have published recommendations on the indications for the use and efficacy targets of lipoprotein apheresis in 2008 and 2010, respectively, and, most recently, on the management of homozygous FH.[13] Members of HEART UK have also participated in drawing up NICE guidelines on lipid modification, the use of ezetimibe, and the identification and management of FH. Important research contributions have also come from the affiliated

Simon Broome Familial Hyperlipidaemia Register, which has produced several major publications since 1998 on the risks of CHD in FH and the benefits of treatment.

Tenth Anniversary of Brown and Goldstein's Nobel Prize

Oliver's commentary after WOSCOPS was entitled "Statins prevent coronary heart disease,"[14] but he remained reluctant to draw any conclusions about non-cardiac mortality, opting to wait for the results of the Heart Protection Study, still several years hence. However, he relented sooner than that at a meeting held in Stockholm in 1996 to celebrate the tenth anniversary of the award of the Nobel Prize to Goldstein and Brown (Figure 2). It was there that he finally completed his U-turn, which he justified by citing Maynard Keynes: "When the facts change, I change my mind. What do you do?"

During the anniversary meeting, Michael Brown gave an after-dinner speech during which he related a story that he'd told in front of the Queen

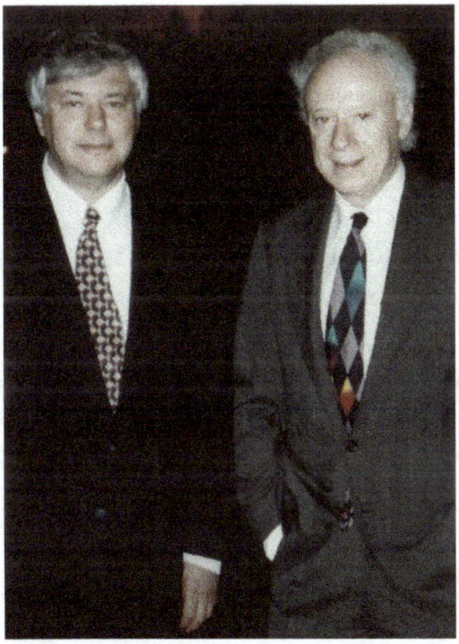

Figure 2. Michael Brown and Joseph Goldstein at the 10th anniversary celebration of their Nobel Prize in Stockholm.

of Sweden on the occasion of the Nobel dinner 10 years previously. It concerned a Nobel laureate who had stopped to fill up at a roadside garage in a small town somewhere in the USA. The laureate's wife recognised the petrol attendant and getting out of the car she went over and warmly embraced him. When she returned to the car she was confronted by her furious husband. "What the hell do you think you're doing kissing that jerk?" "I'm sorry darling" she replied, "but he was my first sweetheart and my feelings all came back in a rush when I recognised him. We were very much in love in those days, so much so that we nearly got married. I sincerely apologise for getting carried away like that." Somewhat mollified, the Nobel Prize winner said "Just as well you didn't marry him or you would never have done all the things we've done together since I became a Nobel laureate." "If I'd married him" retorted his wife, "he'd have got the Nobel Prize, not you!"

Heart Protection Study

Several other statin trials were published between 1995 and 1998, but the largest of them was not completed until the start of the new millennium. This was the Heart Protection Study (HPS), which was designed and conducted by the Oxford-based Clinical Trials Service Unit, with Rory Collins (since knighted) as the principal investigator.[15] This trial examined the effects on mortality and morbidity of cholesterol-lowering therapy in more than 20,000 subjects with, or at high risk of, cardiovascular disease in the UK. Men and women aged 40–80 with serum total cholesterol over 3.5 mmol/l were randomized to receive either simvastatin 40 mg daily or anti-oxidant vitamins, the two combined, or placebo.

The results showed an incidence of major coronary events in those on placebo of 11.8% over 5 years, confirming that they were a high-risk group. Subjects allocated to simvastatin had a mean reduction in LDL cholesterol of 1 mmol/l, with decreases in total and cardiovascular mortality of 12% and 17% and decreases in coronary events and strokes of 26% and 27%, respectively. Benefit from simvastatin occurred irrespective of the level of LDL cholesterol at entry to the study, and was not influenced by age, gender, or clinical status, and there was no increase in non-cardiovascular mortality. One-third of the patients in the HPS had a baseline LDL cholesterol under 3 mmol/l, an important finding suggesting that high-risk individuals (e.g. diabetics) benefit from LDL-lowering even if their LDL cholesterol is considered to be "normal."

Cholesterol Treatment Trialists' Collaboration Meta-analysis

The final dotting of the *i*'s and crossing of the *t*'s that marked the end of the controversy over the lipid hypothesis came when data from over 90,000 individuals who participated in 14 statin trials between 1994 and 2004 were subjected to meta-analysis by the Cholesterol Treatment Trialists' Collaboration (CTTC).[16] The results showed decreases of 12% and 19% in total and coronary mortality, respectively, for each 1 mmol/l reduction in LDL cholesterol, similar to what was found in the HPS. Overall, the risk of a major vascular event, including strokes, was reduced by one-fifth. No significant changes in non-cardiovascular mortality occurred over the 5-year duration of these trials, and one feels that even McMichael would have been convinced. He had previously stated that "All trials of prophylactic measures based on hypotheses of causation have to be examined in the prevention of progression of the disorder in known patients at risk with proven clinical manifestations." The regression trials, together with 4S, HPS, and the CTTC meta-analysis fulfilled his demands and unequivocally proved the validity of the lipid hypothesis. Subsequent trials where more potent statins reduced LDL cholesterol by over 50% have reinforced that verdict.

Wellcome Witness Twentieth Century Medicine Seminar

In 2005, a *Wellcome Witness Seminar on Cholesterol, Atherosclerosis and Coronary Disease in the UK, 1950–2000,* was held at the Wellcome Trust Centre in London. As the title suggests the purpose of the seminar was to hear from those in the UK who had participated in research on that topic during the last 50 years of the 20th century. Sadly, many of them have since died including both Michael Oliver (Figure 1 of Chapter 11), who chaired the meeting and Chris Booth (Figure 3) who, wearing his distinguished

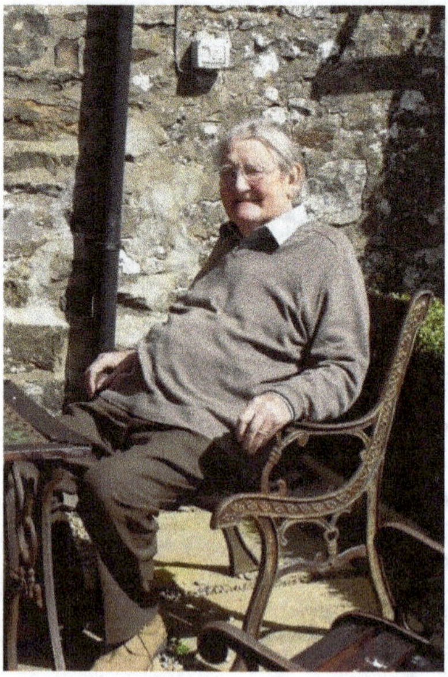

Figure 3. Sir Christopher Booth (1924–2012) in the garden of his cottage in Wensleydale.

medical historian's hat, summed up the proceedings at the end of the day by noting that coronary atherosclerosis was a British disease, first described in 1776 by the surgeon John Hunter.[17] The collective efforts in the past of those who attended the meeting have contributed significantly to elucidating the pathogenesis and treatment of this, the commonest cause of death among men in the UK.

References

1. Thompson GR. Angiographic trials of lipid-lowering therapy: End of an era? *Br Heart J* 1995;**74**:343–7.
2. Buchwald H, Varco RL, Matts JP *et al.* Effect of partial ileal bypass surgery on mortality and morbidity from coronary heart disease in patients with hypercholesterolemia. *N Engl J Med* 1990;**323**:946–55.
3. Brown G, Alberts JJ, Fisher LD. Regression of coronary artery disease as a result of intensive lipid-lowering therapy in men with high levels of apolipoprotein B. *N Engl J Med* 1990;**323**:1289–98.

4. Watts GF, Lewis B, Brunt JNH *et al.* Effects on coronary artery disease of lipid-lowering diet, or diet plus cholestyramine in the St. Thomas' Atherosclerosis Regression Study (STARS). *Lancet* 1992;**339**:563–9.
5. Brown BG, Zhao X-Q, Sacco DE, Albers JJ. Atherosclerosis regression, plaque disruption, and cardiovascular events. A rationale for lipid lowering in coronary artery disease. *Annu Rev Med* 1993;**44**:365–76.
6. Davies MJ, Krikler DM, Katz D. Atherosclerosis: Inhibition or regression as therapeutic possibilities. *Br Heart J* 1991;**65**:302–10.
7. Scandinavian Simvastatin Survival Study Group. Randomised trial of cholesterol lowering in 4444 patients with coronary heart disease: The Scandinavian Simvastatin Survival Study (4S). *Lancet* 1994;**344**:1383–9.
8. Oliver M, Poole-Wilson P, Shepherd J, Tikkanen M. Lower patients' cholesterol now. *Br Med J* 1995;**310**:1280–1.
9. Report from the Committee of Principal Investigators. A co-operative trial in the primary prevention of ischaemic heart disease using clofibrate. *Br Heart J* 1978;**40**:1069–118.
10. Report of the Committee of Principal Investigators. W.H.O. Cooperative trial on primary prevention of ischaemic heart disease using clofibrate to lower serum cholesterol: Mortality follow up. *Lancet* 1980;**2**:379–85.
11. Shepherd J, Cobbe SM, Ford I *et al.* Prevention of coronary heart disease with pravastatin in men with hypercholesterolemia. West of Scotland Coronary Prevention Study Group. *N Engl J Med* 1995;**333**:1301–7.
12. Packard C. Cholesterol, atherosclerosis and coronary disease in the UK, 1950–2000. In Reynolds LA, Tansey EM (eds.), *Wellcome Witnesses to Twentieth Century Medicine*, Vol. 27, 2006, p. 77.
13. France M, Rees A, Datta D *et al.* HEART UK statement on the management of homozygous familial hypercholesterolaemia in the United Kingdom. *Atherosclerosis* 2016;**255**:128–39.
14. Oliver MF. Statins prevent coronary heart disease. *Lancet* 1995;**346**:1378–9.
15. Heart Protection Study Collaborative Group. MRC/BHF heart protection study of cholesterol lowering with simvastatin in 20536 high-risk individuals: A randomised placebo-controlled trial. *Lancet* 2002;**360**:7–22.
16. Baigent C, Keech A, Kearney PM *et al.* Efficacy and safety of cholesterol-lowering treatment: Prospective meta-analysis of data from 90,056 participants in 14 randomised trials of statins. *Lancet* 2005;**366**:1267–78.
17. Booth C. Cholesterol, atherosclerosis and coronary disease in the UK, 1950–2000. In Reynolds LA, Tansey EM (eds.), *Wellcome Witnesses to Twentieth Century Medicine*, Vol. 27, 2006, p. 80.

13 Apheresis — The Cholesterol Take-Away Procedure

Significance of Lipoprotein Apheresis

At this juncture I will pause my narrative in order to discuss whether the introduction of apheresis to remove cholesterol-carrying lipoproteins from the bloodstream constituted a significant advance in clinical practice. Inevitably, this involves the use of technical terms and concepts unfamiliar to some and needing explanation. Starting with apheresis, the word is derived from the Greek "take away" and is a generic term that embraces plasmapheresis, plasma exchange, and lipoprotein apheresis. In contrast to plasmapheresis and plasma exchange, which are unselective procedures, lipoprotein apheresis selectively removes LDL and other apoB-containing particles from the circulation but conserves the remainder of the plasma proteins including HDL, which theoretically is advantageous.

History and Development

Extracorporeal removal of cholesterol to treat homozygous FH was first used over a prolonged period by de Gennes and colleagues in Paris in 1967.[1] They undertook the laborious process of manual plasmapheresis (removing successive pints of blood, centrifuging them, discarding the plasma, and returning the red cells to the patient) repetitively for 4 months. This lowered the patient's serum cholesterol but was abandoned because of his fatigue and that of his physicians. Subsequently, centrifugal cell separators that continuously separated plasma from blood cells were developed in the USA and my colleagues and I used one of these devices, an Aminco Celltrifuge, to undertake plasma exchange in the Haematology department at the Hammersmith. The stimulus to do so arose from the presentation on the Staff Round in 1974 of a patient with macroglobulinaemia (an excess of an abnormally large plasma protein that increases blood viscosity) who was being treated successfully with plasma exchange. The potential of this procedure for removing other proteins present in excess in plasma, such as LDL, was immediately apparent and we soon exploited it, as described earlier. Almost simultaneously, Keith Peters and his colleagues started using apheresis to treat patients with Goodpasture's syndrome (autoantibody-mediated renal disease).[2] Neither of us could have undertaken plasma exchange however, without the provision by the Blood Transfusion Service of supplies of human albumin solution. This was heat-treated and free from the risk of transmitting hepatitis viruses and HIV but the subsequent outbreak of mad cow disease in Britain raised fears that the prion responsible, which is heat resistant, could be transmitted by this route. Consequently, since 1999, human albumin has been imported at considerable cost from countries free from mad cow disease, such as the USA. Lipoprotein apheresis has now largely replaced plasma exchange in the treatment of homozygous FH, eliminating the need for albumin replacements, but plasma exchange is still used to treat other disorders and is currently under investigation for the management of patients with Alzheimer's Disease.

Selective LDL apheresis was first introduced by Stoffel *et al.*[3] in 1981, who used a cell separator to perfuse plasma through an immunoadsorbent column and then return the LDL-depleted plasma to the patient. This procedure has since been largely superseded by methods involving perfusion of plasma or whole blood through affinity columns containing either dextran sulphate covalently linked to cellulose beads or polyacrylate-coated polyacrylamide beads.[4] Similarly to immunoapheresis these bind the apoB component of LDL and lipoprotein(a) (Lp(a) (another risk factor for cardiovascular disease, as described below) and thus remove both these lipoproteins and their cargo of cholesterol from the circulation.

Other approaches to lipoprotein apheresis involve extracorporeal precipitation of LDL through the addition of heparin to plasma, the so-called HELP system, and double filtration plasmapheresis (DFPP), in which plasma is first separated from blood cells by a hollow membrane filter and then perfused through a second filter which selectively retains smaller plasma components like HDL and albumin but discards larger ones, including LDL and Lp(a). Dextran sulphate-based haemoperfusion or plasma adsorption systems are probably the most popular. They are remarkably safe and are also more compact and portable than the centrifugal system that we used for plasma exchange.

Japanese companies were at the forefront of the development of devices used in lipoprotein apheresis and a number of research fellows came over from Japan to work with me during the 1980s and 1990s. With their help we compared the efficacy and tolerability of plasma exchange and lipoprotein apheresis, using the dextran sulphate adsorption system developed by the Japanese company Kaneka. On Christmas Day we used to invite them and their wives to dinner at our house, which we celebrated in traditional style with a turkey and all the trimmings. One Christmas my wife caused confusion among our polite guests when she mistakenly passed them a dish of what she thought was cranberry jelly but which turned out to be raw turkey liver! This caused great hilarity and became part of our family's joke lore.

Objectives of Apheresis

Our initial objective of using plasma exchange was to arrest progression or even induce regression of atherosclerosis in FH homozygotes by reducing their very high cholesterol levels in an attempt to prolong their lives. Untreated, most of these patients died from cardiovascular disease before the age of 30. In 1985, I was deputed by Keith Peters to demonstrate the encouraging results of a decade of plasma exchange on the survival of homozygotes[5] to Her Majesty The Queen when she visited the Royal Postgraduate Medical School on its 50th anniversary (Figure 1). However, final proof that the procedure increased longevity did not come until 2018 when, together with colleagues in South Africa, we demonstrated a strong correlation between the total mortality of FH homozygotes and their level of cholesterol on treatment, the latter reflecting the combined effects of apheresis and lipid-lowering drugs (see Chapter 18).

Another of our objectives was to investigate whether the reduced rate of removal of LDL from plasma in untreated FH patients was a primary phenomenon reflecting their lack of LDL receptors, which had recently been discovered by Goldstein and Brown,[6] or due to saturation of the removal pathway by an expanded LDL pool. By measuring LDL turnover before and after plasma exchange we were able to show that LDL removal

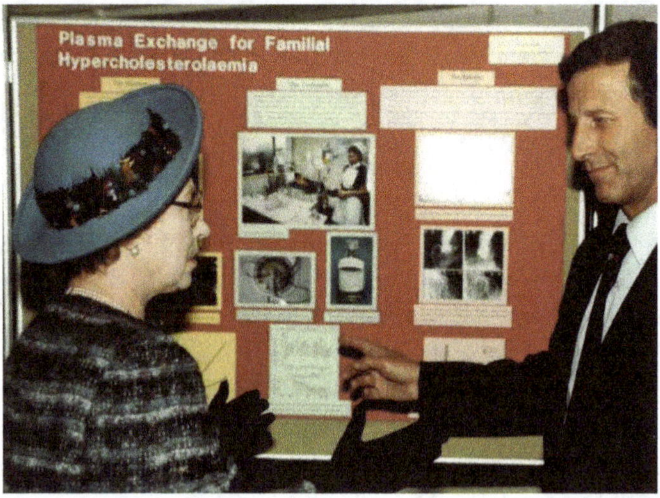

Figure 1. Demonstrating the results of plasma exchange to Her Majesty the Queen in 1985.

was subnormal in FH patients prior to plasma exchange, especially in homozygotes, and that it remained subnormal even after their enlarged LDL pool had been lowered to normal by plasma exchange; this supported the existence of an intrinsic clearance defect.[7] Our results were in keeping with Goldstein and Brown's discovery that partial and total absence of LDL receptors were the cause of heterozygous and homozygous FH, respectively.[8] Their studies involved measuring the saturable uptake of radioactive LDL by cultured fibroblasts (skin cells) from normal subjects *in vitro* and demonstrating its absence in fibroblasts from a patient with homozygous FH. Our clinical observations supported their laboratory findings and led to invitations to give seminars at the NIH and to their own department at the University of Texas Southwestern Medical School in Dallas.

A Surrogate LDL Receptor

The original rationale for using apheresis to treat homozygous FH is epitomised by a well-known quotation from Shakespeare's *Hamlet*: "Diseases desperate grown, by desperate appliance are relieved, or not at all." Homozygous FH was and still is a desperate disease requiring radical therapy to prevent its often catastrophic consequences. However, apheresis is not simply a desperate manoeuvre without any scientific basis. The extreme hypercholesterolaemia of homozygous FH is largely due to the absence of LDL receptors in the liver, which are the main determinants of LDL cholesterol levels in the blood. LDL catabolism (removal) is governed by first-order kinetics, which means that the fractional rate of removal of LDL remains constant irrespective of LDL pool size. The absence of LDL receptors results in a reduction of receptor-mediated catabolism of LDL and hence to a greatly expanded pool. By physically removing LDL, apheresis acts as a surrogate LDL receptor in patients who lack them and because the rate of production of LDL obeys zero order kinetics (i.e. remains constant irrespective of pool size), apheresis enhances the removal of LDL from plasma without increasing its rate of production.

The magnitude of the acute reduction in LDL following apheresis depends upon the volume of plasma or whole blood that is treated. An acute decrease to 70% below the baseline is achieved by treating 1.2 plasma volumes (3.75 L in a 70-kg person). Subsequently, there is an exponential rebound in the plasma level of LDL, which gradually plateaus to reach its baseline value after about 40 days in FH homozygotes, 20 days in heterozygotes and 10 days in normal subjects (Figure 2). These differences reflect differences in their respective fractional catabolic rates (FCR) of LDL, which average roughly 0.1, 0.2, and 0.4 pools per day. The lower the FCR the

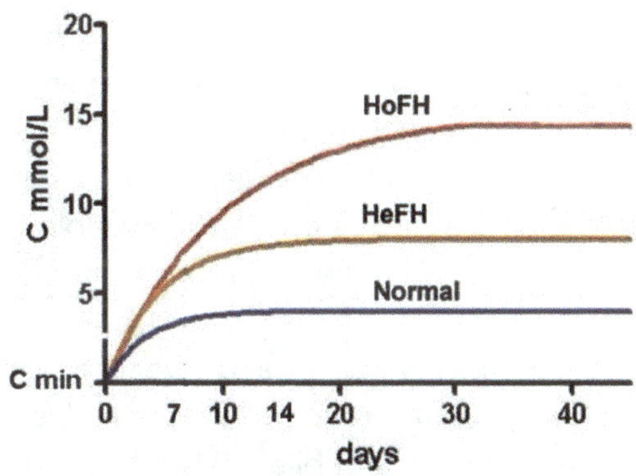

Figure 2. Rebounds in plasma cholesterol (C) from post-apheresis values (C min) are illustrated in a normal subject, FH heterozygote (HeFH), and FH homozygote (HoFH).

larger the pool size must be before the rate of removal equals the rate of production of LDL and a steady state is reached. The FCR of an individual can be determined by calculating the first order disappearance constant of their post-apheresis rebound in LDL, as described by Apstein *et al.*[9]

Because the post-apheresis rebound in LDL is curvilinear, the best estimate of the ensuing reduction in LDL is obtained by calculating the interval mean value (the area under the rebound curve divided by time) of LDL cholesterol between successive procedures. From a pragmatic viewpoint, weekly apheresis is acceptable to most FH homozygotes and gives a 46% reduction in the interval mean LDL cholesterol from its baseline value. Concomitant administration of a statin and ezetimibe decreases this further to 70% below the baseline. Although the main consequence of apheresis is to reduce the concentration of LDL cholesterol in the circulation, there is some evidence that it also promotes influx of HDL cholesterol by stimulating the process known as reverse cholesterol transport.

Effect on Cholesterol Turnover in the Body

The impact of apheresis on the turnover of LDL cholesterol within the circulation is reflected by its subsequent effect on the transport of cholesterol to and from the rest of the body, including the arterial wall. By measuring the turnover of ^{14}C-cholesterol for up to 10 months after its intravenous administration to normal and hyperlipidaemic subjects and, based on the differing rates of equilibration of labelled with unlabelled cholesterol, Goodman *et al.*[10] proposed the existence of 3 physiological pools of cholesterol: Pool 1, the rapidly exchangeable pool, represents the cholesterol in plasma lipoproteins, red blood cells, liver, intestines, and other organs; Pool 2, with an intermediate rate of exchange, represents cholesterol in skin and adipose tissue; and Pool 3, the slowly exchangeable pool, represents cholesterol in skeletal muscle and the arterial wall (Figure 3).

Under steady-state conditions the input of cholesterol into pool 1 from synthesis, mainly by the liver, plus that derived from intestinal absorption of dietary cholesterol, totals roughly 1 g/day and is balanced by its output as faecal neutral sterols and bile acids. Most turnover studies in FH patients have shown rates of cholesterol and bile acid synthesis that are within the normal range.[11] However, raised plasma cholesterol levels in

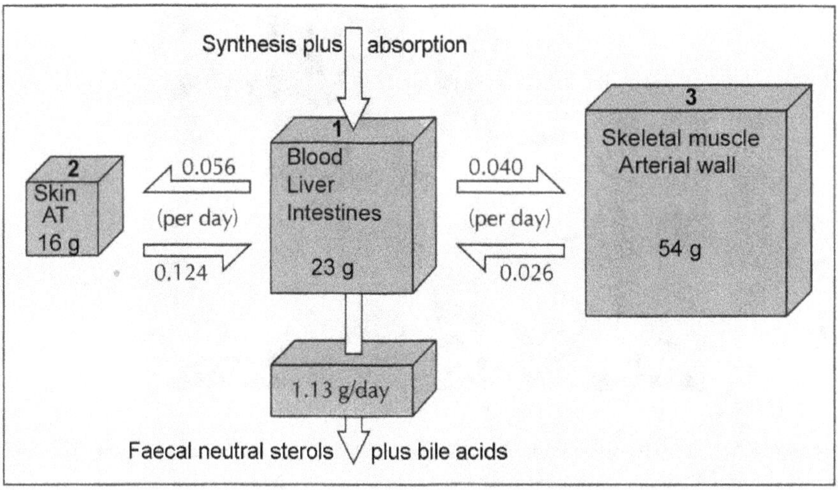

Figure 3. Three pool model of cholesterol turnover in humans (based on data from Ref. 10). Pool (1) rapidly exchangeable; (2) intermediate rate of exchange; (3) slowly exchangeable. The mass of cholesterol in each pool and fractional transfer rates between them are shown (AT in pool 2 = adipose tissue).

FH, due to defective clearance of LDL, will expand the size of pool 1 and consequently the mass of cholesterol transported from pool 1 to pools 2 and 3 is increased in patients with untreated FH. This is manifested clinically by cutaneous and tendon xanthomas and by the severity of aortic and coronary atherosclerosis in homozygotes.

The slowest of the fractional transfer rates of cholesterol is from pool 3 to 1, which represents the average of the very different rates of efflux of cholesterol from skeletal muscle and the arterial wall; Jagannathan *et al.*[12] showed that the turnover of cholesterol in atheromatous plaques in the aorta and coronary arteries is 10 times slower than in skeletal muscle. Furthermore, Katz *et al.*[13] found that the rate of turnover of cholesterol within an atheromatous plaque varies according to its physical state and location, the turnover of crystalline free cholesterol in the depth of the lesion being much slower than that of the cholesterol, mainly esterified (i.e. covalently linked to a fatty acid), in the remainder of the plaque. Cholesterol crystals comprise up to 40% of the free cholesterol in atheromatous plaques and are especially prominent in FH homozygotes, which suggests that mobilisation of cholesterol would be especially slow in this situation.

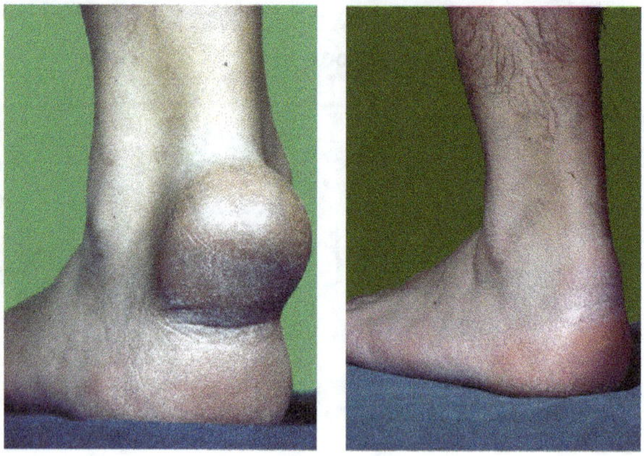

Figure 4. Achilles tendon xanthoma of patient with homozygous familial hypercholesterolaemia before and after 6 years of plasma exchange.

Unfortunately, no data exist on the rate of turnover of cholesterol in atheromatous plaques in FH homozygotes. However, we established that it took 6 years of repetitive plasma exchange to achieve total resolution of a golf ball-sized (45 g) Achilles tendon xanthoma in one such patient (Figure 4).[14] Assuming it had a cholesterol content of 30 g and knowing that plasmapheresis removed 100 g of plasma cholesterol each year, the estimated turnover of xanthoma cholesterol was 5 g/year or 14 mg/day, one-twentieth of the rate at which cholesterol was removed from plasma by apheresis. Given that the turnover rates of cholesterol in tendons and the arterial wall are similar,[13] one can speculate that apheresis mobilises cholesterol from atheromatous plaques and tendon xanthomas at comparable rates. Figure 2 of Chapter 10 illustrated that significant regression of a presumably cholesterol-rich atheromatous lesion in a coronary artery occurred after only 18 months of lipid-lowering therapy with apheresis and a statin.

Recently published clinical data support the premise that cholesterol-lowering measures do indeed have a beneficial effect on the atherosclerotic manifestations of homozygous FH. Atheroma of the aortic root and valve is a particularly severe and potentially lethal complication of the condition but a French study showed that its incidence is greatly reduced if apheresis is started in early childhood.[15] Furthermore, our recent longitudinal survey of UK patients found that the frequency of aortic stenosis in homozygotes treated during the pre-statin era was twice that of those who started treatment after statins became widely available in the 1990s, reflecting greater lowering of serum cholesterol when apheresis and statins are combined.[16]

Effect on Lp(a)

Lp(a) was discovered by Kare Berg,[17] who showed that high levels were inherited and were apparently associated with premature cardiovascular disease (CVD). Subsequently, Mary Seed and her colleagues described an association between raised Lp(a) levels and CVD in FH patients.[18] More recent studies have unequivocally established its role as a causal and independent risk factor.[19] Other studies suggest, but with less certainty, that therapeutic lowering of Lp(a) by apheresis may reduce this risk.

Lp(a) consists of an LDL particle to which is attached a glycoprotein, apolipoprotein(a) or apo(a), covalently linked to the apoB moiety of LDL. The presence of apo(a) greatly reduces the affinity of Lp(a) for the LDL receptor compared with LDL and presumably explains why raised Lp(a) levels in plasma are unaffected by statins, which upregulate LDL receptors. Apo(a) has close structural similarity with plasminogen, which endows Lp(a) with anti-fibrinolytic properties via its competitive inhibition of tissue-type plasminogen activator-mediated activation of plasminogen. Thus, Lp(a) has the potential for promoting both atherosclerosis and thrombosis.

Plasma concentrations of Lp(a) range from 0 to >2000 mg/L and are markedly skewed towards lower values in European populations, 500 mg/L being the 80th percentile. Turnover studies suggest that the assembly of Lp(a) from newly synthesised LDL and apo(a) takes place intracellularly in the liver; the increased production of LDL that we first documented in FH patients may explain why many of them have Lp(a) levels that are two- to three-fold higher than normal subjects.[20] An European Atherosclerosis Society Consensus Panel advised that Lp(a) should be measured in subjects known to be at high risk of CVD, including those with FH and with statin-refractory hypercholesterolaemia and CVD. Values of >500 mg/L are regarded as undesirably high.[21]

Currently, the only effective means of reducing Lp(a) levels is by undertaking weekly lipoprotein apheresis. Recently, an analysis of the German Lipoprotein Apheresis Registry for the period 2012–2015 reported that acute reductions of both LDL-cholesterol and Lp(a) averaged approximately 70% in patients undergoing apheresis.[22] The data also showed a dramatic reduction (−97%) in cardiovascular events when their occurrence during the period before initiation of apheresis was compared with the period following institution of regular apheresis. Randomized controlled trial data are lacking but should soon become available now that novel compounds that drastically lower Lp(a) by interfering with the translation of apo(a) RNA are undergoing clinical testing.[23]

Past and Future Use of Lipoprotein Apheresis

This summary of the evidence suggests that the opportunistic use of plasma exchange to treat homozygous FH in the 1970s did indeed provide a safe and effective means of ameliorating a previously untreatable disorder. It also paved the way for selective lipoprotein apheresis and provided important data on the non-steady-state kinetics of LDL and the turnover of cholesterol in tendon xanthomas in FH and therefore, by extrapolation, in atheromatous plaques. It further provided an effective means of reducing raised levels of Lp(a). Lastly and most importantly, it helped establish that the frequency of cardiovascular events and survival of FH homozygotes are determined by the level to which their LDL cholesterol is lowered when apheresis is combined with drug treatment. In an email to me, Mike Brown referred to this finding and wrote, "you and your colleagues ... have extended many lives."

The recent advent of the novel LDL-lowering drug lomitapide has already reduced the number of FH homozygotes needing apheresis. However, it is probable that there will always be a small number of patients, especially children and pregnant women, in whom apheresis is the only safe and effective LDL-lowering option. Furthermore, as already discussed, it is currently the sole form of treatment available for patients with CVD due to raised levels of Lp(a).[4] Apheresis may be past its prime but for the time being it still has an important therapeutic role.

References

1. de Gennes J-L, Touraine R, Maunand B *et al. Formes homozygotes cutane-tendineuses de xanthomatose hypercholésterolémique dans une observation familiale exemplaire. Essai de plasmaphérése à titre de traitment héroique. Bull Mem Soc Hop Paris* 1967;**118**:252–4.
2. Lockwood CM, Boulton-Jones JM, Lowenthal RM, Simpson IJ, Peters DK. Recovery from Goodpasture's syndrome after immunosuppressive treatment and plasmapheresis. *Br Med J* 1975;**ii**:252–4.
3. Stoffel W, Borberg H, Greve V. Application of specific extracorporeal removal of low density lipoprotein in familial hypercholesterolaemia. *Lancet* 1981;**2**:1005–7.
4. Thompson G, Parhofer K. Current role of lipoprotein apheresis. *Curr Atherosclerosis Reports* 2019;**21**:26, https://doi.org/10.1007/s11883-019-0787-5.
5. Thompson GR, Miller JP, Breslow JL. Improved survival of patients with homozygous familial hypercholesterolaemia treated with plasma exchange. *Br Med J* 1985;**291**:1671–3.
6. Goldstein JL, Brown MS. Familial hypercholesterolemia: Identification of a defect in the regulation of 3-hydroxy-3-methylglutaryl coenzyme A reductase activity associated with overproduction of cholesterol. *Proc Natl Acad Sci USA* 1973;**70**:2804–8.
7. Thompson GR, Spinks T, Ranicar A, Myant NB. Non-steady state studies of low-density lipoprotein turnover in familial hypercholesterolaemia. *Clin Sci Mol Med* 1977;**52**:361–9.
8. Goldstein JL, Brown MS. Binding and degradation of low density lipoproteins by cultured human fibroblasts. *J Biol Chem* 1974;**249**:5153–62.
9. Apstein CS, Zilversmit DB, Lees RS, George PK. Effect of intensive plasmapheresis on the plasma cholesterol concentration with familial hypercholesterolemia. *Atherosclerosis* 1978;**31**:105–15.
10. Goodman DS, Noble RP, Dell RB. Three-pool model of the long-term turnover of plasma cholesterol in man. *J Lipid Res* 1973;**14**:178–88.
11. Myant NB. *The Biology of Cholesterol and Related Steroids.* London: William Heinemann Medical Books Ltd; 1981.
12. Jagannathan SN, Connor WE, Baker WH, A. K. Bhattacharrya AK. The Turnover of Cholesterol in Human Atherosclerotic Arteries. *J Clin Invest* 1974;**54**:366–77.
13. Katz SS, Small DM, Smith FR, Dell RB, Goodman DS. Cholesterol turnover in lipid phases of human atherosclerotic plaque. *J Lipid Res* 1982;**23**:733–7.

14. Thompson GR, Barbir M, Okabayashi K, Trayner I, Larkin S. Plasmapheresis in familial hypercholesterolemia. *Arteriosclerosis*. 1989;**9**(Suppl 1):1152–7.
15. Lefort B, Saheb S, Bruckert E, Giraud C, Hequet O, Hankard R. Impact of LDL apheresis on aortic root atheroma in children with homozygous familial hypercholesterolemia. *Atherosclerosis* 2015;**239**:158–62.
16. Thompson GR, Seed M, Naoumova RP *et al.* Improved cardiovascular outcomes following temporal advances in lipid-lowering therapy in a genetically-characterised cohort of familial hypercholesterolaemia homozygotes. *Atherosclerosis*. 2015;**243**:328–33.
17. Berg K, Mohr J. Genetics of the Lp system. *Acta Genet* 1963;**13**:349–60.
18. Seed M, Hoppichler F, Reaveley D, *et al.* Relation of serum lipoprotein(a) concentration and apolipoprotein(a) phenotype to coronary heart disease in patients with familial hypercholesterolemia. *N Eng J Med* 1990;**322**:1494–99.
19. Kronenberg F, Utermann G. Lipoprotein(a): Resurrected by genetics. *J Intern Med* 2013;**273**:6–30.
20. Soutar AK, Myant NB, Thompson GR. Simultaneous measurement of apolipoprotein B turnover in very low and low density lipoproteins in familial hypercholesterolaemia. *Atherosclerosis* 1977;**28**:247–56.
21. Nordestgaard BG, Chapman MJ, Ray K *et al.* Lipoprotein(a) as a cardiovascular risk factor: Current status. *Eur Ht J* 2010;**31**:2844–53.
22. Schettler VJ, Neumann CL, Peter C *et al.* The German lipoprotein apheresis registry (GLAR) — almost 5 years on. *Clin Res Cardiol Suppl* 2017;**12**(Suppl 1): 44–9.
23. Tsimikas S, Viney NJ, Hughes SG, Singleton W *et al.* Antisense therapy targeting apolipoprotein(a): A randomised, double-blind, placebo-controlled phase 1 study. *Lancet* 2015;**386**:1472–83.

14 Scotland

Knoydart

Fishing provided me with an opportunity to get away from work for a week or two each summer and of all the places in Scotland I've been to in search of salmon, the loveliest is Knoydart. It combines rustic simplicity with rugged grandeur, the cluster of cottages fringing Inverie Bay contrasting with the mountains that form their backdrop and are the source of Knoydart's rivers. I first went there in 1979 when, thanks to its remoteness, it was a little-known and totally unspoilt part of Scotland. That was the year after the Winter of Discontent when the Labour Prime Minister, James Callaghan, lost a vote of confidence in the House of Commons. The ensuing general election resulted in a Conservative victory and the installation of Margaret Thatcher as Britain's first female Prime Minister.

Knoydart comprises a peninsula on the west coast of Inverness-shire, separated from the southern tip of the Isle of Skye by the Sound of Sleat (Figure 1). It is accessible from the Scottish mainland only by boat or on foot, the nearest approach roads for motor vehicles terminating at Kinloch Hourn on Loch Hourn to the northeast or petering out at Glendessary, several miles short of Loch Nevis in the southeast. However, there is a short stretch of road on Knoydart itself running from Inverie, the main settlement, to Inverguseran at the mouth of the Guseran River on the Sound of Sleat. The first time I took my car over there from Mallaig I watched nervously while it was loaded by crane onto a converted wartime landing craft owned by the Estate and called the Spanish John. On arrival at Inverie, I had to drive down the ramps of the landing craft into the water and then up the pebble beach, rather like a Jeep on D Day. This was quite tricky because

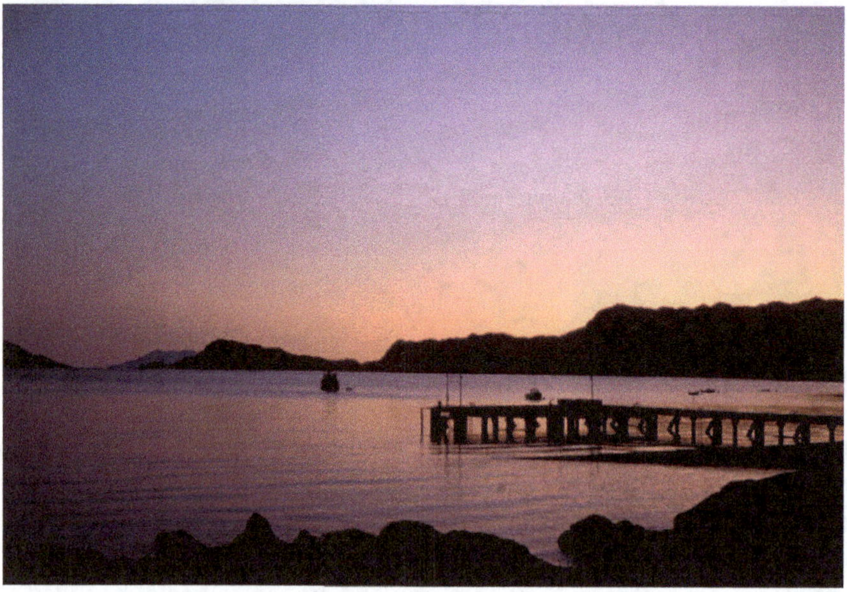

Figure 1. Sunset over Inverie harbour, Knoydart.

it was not a Jeep but a rear wheel drive BMW, this being long before the advent of four wheel drive versions of the latter.

Currently, the resident adult population of Knoydart consists of roughly a hundred persons but it was 10 times that number in the 1850s, prior to the Highland clearances. Many of the crofters who were evicted emigrated to Canada. In 1999, after a long period of private ownership, the Estate was bought by and is now managed by the Knoydart Foundation, a partnership of local residents and charitable trusts.

The Inverie and the Guseran

During the summers that I was there Knoydart was a paradise for fishermen and hill walkers. The main salmon and sea trout rivers are the Inverie and Guseran, both of which I fished with a split cane trout rod that soon developed a permanent bend. The salmon were not especially big but the sea trout ran up to 6 lb and fought like tigers. To get to the Guseran

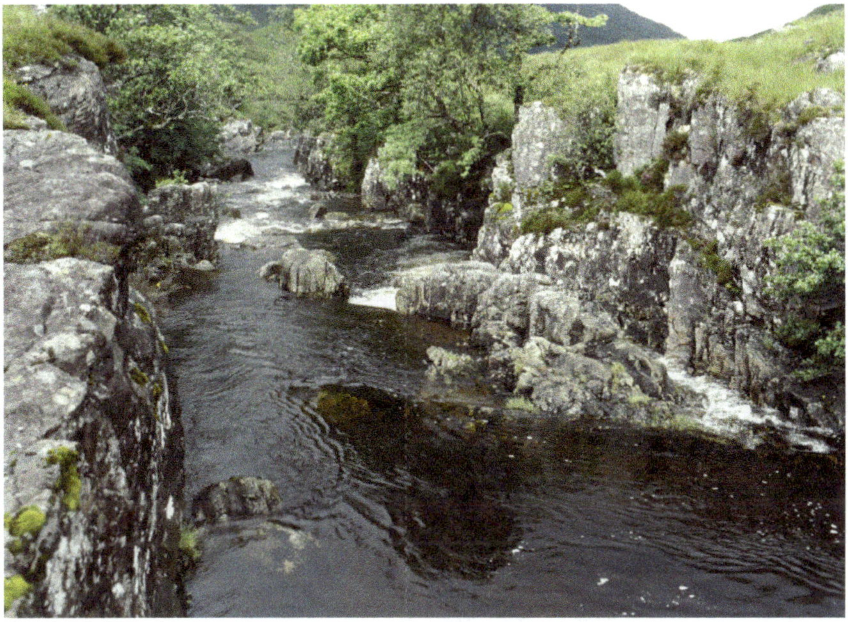

Figure 2. Guseran River, Knoydart.

involved driving or walking along a track for several miles. Once there one had to be prepared for some athletic fishing, which involved scrambling along the top of the ravine in which the turbulent river ran and around trees sprouting from the rocks if one was to prevent a hooked sea trout returning to the Sound of Sleat whence it came (Figure 2). The Inverie was a more peaceful and accessible river, originating in Loch Dubh Lochan and emptying into Inverie Bay, but it too had sizeable sea trout as well as good runs of grilse and salmon.

On one occasion, when the water level in the Inverie was low and the salmon were dour one of my fellow guests, who was French, was casting half in jest with his trout rod at a salmon that was lying behind a large boulder. Failing to get a response he waded out to the front of the boulder and dapped a fly right over the salmon's nose. This irritated the fish so much that it grabbed the fly then tore off downstream, snapping the thin trout cast in the process. The Frenchman got full marks from the rest of us for initiative if not for execution.

Munros

Another alternative on hot, dry days was to head for the hills. For Munro baggers Knoydart is the home of four 3,000 footers, Ladhar Bheinn, Luinne Bheinn, Meall Buidhe, and Sgùrr na Cìche. The first three are all approached by following the path that goes uphill for 5 miles alongside Loch Dubh Lochan. However, Sgùrr na Cìche (rocky peak of the breast) is far more remote. When approaching Inverie by sea its pointed tip pokes up in the distance like a gun-sight between the shoulders of lower, nearer hills. In terms of proximity, the closest habitation to Sgùrr na Cìche is Camusrory at the top of Loch Nevis but one needs a boat or helicopter to get there.

I resolved to climb this iconic mountain and concluded that it would best be approached from the east, as advised in the Scottish Mountaineering Club's guidebook to the Munros. Thus, in the summer of 1982, I took the road from Fort William to Spean Bridge and then drove along the north bank of Loch Arkaig, parking my car in Upper Glendessary where the road became a track and then ended besides an old wooden shack which had "Path" and an arrow scratched on one of its planks. Laden with a tent and provisions I hiked westwards in the direction of the arrow until I reached the banks of a stream, where I camped for the night. This was the area where some of Bonnie Prince Charlie's Jacobite supporters, and possibly the Prince himself, hid out after their disastrous defeat by Loyalist troops under the command of the Duke of Cumberland at Culloden in 1746.

The following day, taking my fishing rod with me on what proved to be a fruitless quest for a trout in one of the higher lochans, I climbed to the top of Sgùrr na Cìche in perfect weather and was rewarded with spectacular views. To the west were the mountains that form the "Rough Bounds of Knoydart," Loch Quoich slanted north-eastwards below me; and to the east, in the distance, was the snow clad bulk of Ben Nevis. The only other person on top of Sgùrr na Cìche was slightly bemused by my fishing rod, not standard Munro equipment, but we shook hands and took each other's photos. Mission accomplished, I descended the mountain to find the tent and the car both intact and the sun still shining. I was hot, thirsty, and triumphant — until I discovered there was no beer left with which to cool off.

On my last visit to Knoydart, which was in 1984, I decided to take the train to Mallaig from Fort William rather than drive as on previous occasions.

I was sitting in my carriage and enjoying the scenery when the train stopped unexpectedly a few miles short of Mallaig. No explanation was given as to why but as time went by I grew increasingly restless since I needed to get to Mallaig in time to catch the Estate boat to Inverie. So I jumped off the train, carrying all my gear and made my way to the adjacent road with the intention of hitchhiking to Mallaig. This was easier said than done, initially proving fruitless despite my best efforts, which included waving a £10 note at passing motorists as I walked along the road. Eventually, just as I was getting desperate, an open-topped convertible stopped and the driver kindly offered me a lift. I got the impression that he might have been a pop musician and fisherman, possibly a well-known one, but I never discovered his identity. However, thanks to him I got to Inverie and I raised my glass to him that evening in the Old Forge, the only pub in Knoydart.

The highlight of my stay came on the last night when at 11:30 pm, 4 hours after high tide, I caught a sea trout in the Sea Pool of the Inverie. I can still recall the aggressively loud splash the fish made when it rose and the difficulties of casting to it by sound rather than by sight and then having to play and land it, all in near total darkness. It weighed just under 4 lb and, in those pre-catch and release days, I kept it and put it in the freezer when I got back to base, which was well after midnight.

Salmon Farms

I have caught bigger fish than that on the Guseran, a remote little river with water the colour of an Islay malt whisky where one needs Tarzan-like abilities to cope with the sea trout for which it has long been renowned. Hopefully they will continue to run up it, that is unless an accursed fish farm is put near the routes they take through the Sound of Sleat to reach the mouth of the river at Inverguseran. The sea lice that breed on and then are released from these ecological disasters parasitize the wild sea trout and salmon while they are on their way to the rivers of their birth to spawn, thereby decimating their numbers. In the words of the late Bruce Sandison, renowned Scottish angler, journalist, and conservationist, "Salmon farming is an abomination. For the sake of producing fake food we are sacrificing the treasure of the sea. I wouldn't feed it to my cat." His campaign for a ban on sea cages near salmon rivers and for a revolution in fish farming was strongly supported by Orri Vigfússon, who did so much for conservation through his North Atlantic Salmon Fund right up until the time of his recent death.

Unfortunately, these pioneers of salmon conservation have been opposed by strong commercial interests whose sole purpose is to sell as much of their artificially reared salmon as possible to supermarkets and thus to the public at large. A scathing indictment of the supine attitude of the Scottish Government to this situation was published recently by James Merryweather in his article "Truth, lies and fish-farming,"[1] in which he reviews the scientific evidence for the harm done by this vested interest-driven industry in the name of profit, including the huge quantity of organic waste generated by the 250 salmon farms in Scottish waters and their temporal and geographical coincidence with the decline in local populations of wild salmon and sea trout. Instead he proposes the alternative method of closed containment, where the entire process of farming salmon is confined to land-based tanks within which parasites, diseases, and waste are all under complete control, as is happening in Norway. His views chime with Bruce Sandison's, whose key message was a powerful one and worth reiterating: "For the sake of producing fake food we are sacrificing the treasure of the sea." And that is not fake news — the number of salmon caught in Scottish rivers in 2018 was the lowest since records began.

Sutherland

Rivalling Knoydart in terms of its beauty is the western part of the county of Sutherland, with its heather-clad wilderness from which arise dramatic-looking mountains. From the fisherman's point of view the best salmon river, the Helmsdale, is in the eastern part of the county which stretches across Scotland from coast to coast. However, there is a river in the west that runs it close in providing excitement, or did in pre-salmon farm times, namely the Kirkaig.

It was Hermon who first mentioned the Kirkaig to me and waxed eloquent — as only an Irishman can — about the great time he had catching sea trout in the river's estuary near Lochinver. It sounded worth a visit — the only snag was getting there. Lochinver is a small fishing port on the west coast of Sutherland, just north of Ullapool. To reach it from London meant traversing almost the entire length of England and Scotland. This involved driving 670 miles which, on a good day, took 10½ to 11 hours. It's nearly all motorway until Perth, followed by a long slog up the A9 to Inverness. The route then branches off westwards to Ullapool, past the dam at the bottom of Loch Glascarnoch, a man-made reservoir. The final part of the journey is along the road on the north side of Loch Assynt and past the iconic ruin of Ardvreck Castle, which sticks out from the shore like a sore thumb.

Ardvreck was built in the 16th century by the MacLeods, who owned the surrounding lands of Assynt. Its main claim to fame, or perhaps infamy, is that the Marquis of Montrose sought refuge there after the Royalists lost the battle of Carbisdale to the Covenanters. However, instead of being given sanctuary he was handed over to his enemies and taken to Edinburgh, where he was hung, drawn, and quartered in 1650. Subsequently, the castle was captured by the Mackenzies, who commandeered some of the stones from its walls and then allowed it to fall into ruin. If Ardvreck was shrouded in mist and rain on the journey going up, I used to reckon that the omens were good for salmon fishing (Figure 3). But if the sun was shining on

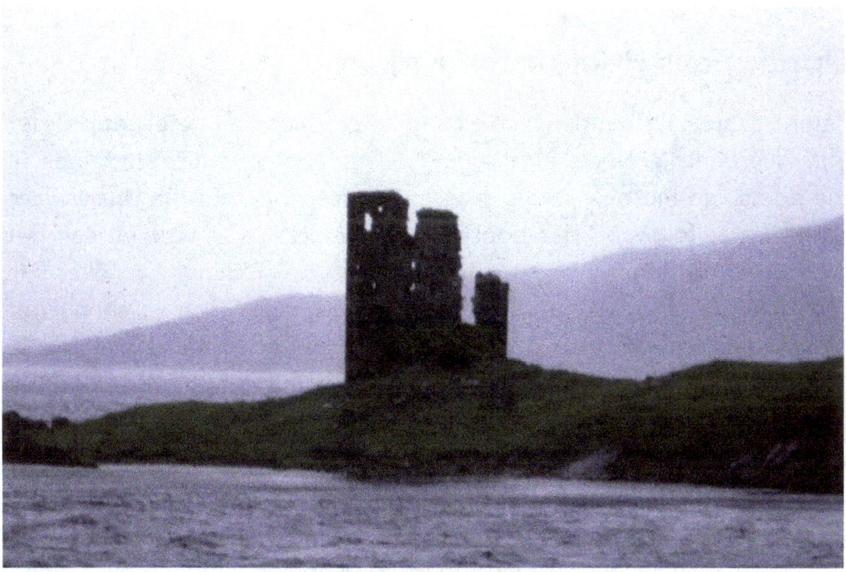

Figure 3. Ardvreck Castle, Sutherland.

Ardvreck, this often meant a week of good weather ahead and having to substitute a camera for a fishing rod.

Lochinver

My first visit to Lochinver was in August 1985 when together with my younger son, aged 14, I stayed for a week at the Culag Hotel. Built at the end of the 18th century as a fish smokery, it was later converted into a summer residence for the Duke of Sutherland. The Gothic-style building is a prominent landmark on the quayside of Lochinver, with the imposing bulk of Suilven forming an impressive backdrop. The plumbing was antiquated but the hot water and drying cupboards were always piping hot.

Salmon fishing for hotel residents was managed in those days by Lorna Hay, wife of Peter Hay, the Factor of the Assynt Estate. Fishing was available on the Inver, upper Oykel, and Kirkaig but the most sought after beats were those on the Kirkaig. The Inver is a more peaceful river than the Kirkaig and has smaller fish whereas the upper beats of the Oykel are so far from the mouth of the river that the fish are black by the time they arrive there.

Upper Falls Pool of the Kirkaig

Peter Hay was a fisherman himself and he produced an excellent booklet *The River Kirkaig. Notes for the guidance of anglers,* which describes all the pools and the best taking places. His description of the Upper Falls pool runs as follows: "This pool holds the most fish as nothing can get any further upstream. Fish once hooked must be held in this pool as it is quite impossible to follow a fish downstream. The Big Falls pool should not be fished unless accompanied by another person, as it requires two people to land a fish. To gaff a fish one slides down to the right hand side of the fishing stance, and onto a ledge. There is a rope attached to the rock as a hand-hold. When gaffed the gaff and fish are handed up to the angler who must take care not to let the fish off the gaff and drop on the head of his ghillie!"

More than 50 years earlier Augustus Grimble[2] described how a friend of his, when fishing the Upper Falls pool, "slipped, fell and bounded from the hard rock with a thud into the horrible, black, boiling pool below. Luckily ... being an extra good swimmer, with a very steady nerve, he came out none the worse: but had he not possessed these qualifications, his chance would indeed have been a poor one." It certainly would.

Full of expectation tinged with slight foreboding, my son and I trudged for a couple of miles up the path from the car park to the top of the river. We were sharing a rod that day on the Upper Falls pool which, as Grimble describes, is an awesome place (Figure 4). Great care has to be taken not to slip when climbing down to the rocky stance where one stands and casts into the pool below and soon gets soaked with spray from the huge waterfall. I fished it first that day but without success. My young son then took the rod and hooked a salmon in the tail of the pool. Mindful of Peter Hay's advice he desperately tried to prevent the fish from going over the sill into the pool below. After half an hour or so he became increasingly exhausted and begged me to take the rod. I refused and told him he must land it or lose it. Alas, the hook came out and the fish got off, to his bitter disappointment.

However, there is a happy ending to this story. Six years later we were fishing the Kirkaig again, this time each of us with his own rod. My son was

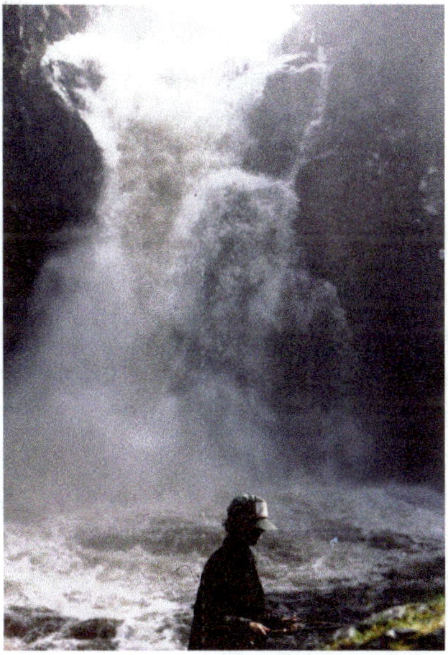

Figure 4. Fishing the Upper Falls Pool, River Kirkaig.

fishing the Upper Falls pool while I was on one of the lower beats. On this occasion he hooked and played a fish successfully but found that landing it was not so easy. It entailed him descending from the fishing stance to the landing ledge at water level, holding on to the rope with one hand, and to his net and rod with the other, all the while trying to keep the line taut. He eventually managed to net the fish but then had to rely on the assistance of an American tourist who'd come to view the Falls, to land it. This involved passing the landing net, fish, and fishing rod up to his helper, which then enabled him to use both hands to climb back onto the fishing stance and claim victory. Peter Hay was right — two people are needed to fish this pool!

Upper Smashie

I fished the Kirkaig on numerous occasions over a period of 12 years, often together with my younger son. From 1988 onwards, this necessitated us staying in the newly-built Inver Lodge hotel instead of the Culag. Both of us enjoyed the physical as well as the piscatorial challenges of the Kirkaig. To quote Augustus Grimble again, "I know of no other river in Scotland which requires such hard walking, so much scrambling and careful placing of feet, as this one. In many places the angler will have to descend and then again ascend very steep rocky banks … and repeat the same process to fish the next pool; the amount of hard work for the legs is out of all proportion to that called for from the arms."

More recently, just before he died, Bruce Sandison wrote, "For me, the upper beat of the River Kirkaig is … 'the salmon river from hell'. It is beyond compare. I don't think that anybody has the right to call themselves a salmon angler until they have tackled this part of the river. It is pure mountain-goat country, from Falls Pool at the top to Arrow Pool at the end."

The truth of those descriptions came home to me with a vengeance in 1994 when my son and I were once again fishing the Kirkaig. I was fishing the pool immediately below the Upper Falls pool, ominously named Upper Smashie. Peter Hay's guide advised trying to find a way down near the head of this pool to avoid disturbing the main lie, which is in the tail. The way down consisted of very steep scree interspersed with small bushes.

On my way down I slipped and reacted by pushing my leg out into the nearest bush to slow my fall, knowing that my son had slipped there previously and smashed his rod. I avoided breaking mine but at the cost, it later transpired, of rupturing the anterior cruciate ligament in my left knee and also getting a salmon fly imbedded in my right thumb, rendering it impossible for me to move. My son, now a medical student, managed to cut the fly out of my thumb with a very blunt penknife and with his help I eventually extricated myself from my predicament and slowly hobbled down the path back to the car park. Upper Smashie had lived up to its name. My knee injury remained undiagnosed until after I had run, rather slowly, in the New York marathon later that year.

Suilven

In contrast to the events described above I recall another occasion with a happier outcome. The weather that day was too good for fishing so I decided instead to climb Suilven, which rises up from the moor through which the Kirkaig winds on its way down to the Falls. By now it was after lunch so I had to get a move on if I was to get there and back before dark. So I set off up the path, passing the lower, middle, and upper beats until I was above the Falls and in sight of Suilven, its primaeval shape reflected in the still surface of a loch in the foreground (Figure 5).

While on my way up to the mountain I saw the astonishing sight of a golden eagle suddenly swoop down from the sky, then reappear from behind a bank of peat with a hare in its claws. As the eagle began to ascend the hare started to kick, and it did this so vigorously that the huge bird eventually dropped its prey and flew off empty handed. An example of Darwin's concept of survival of the fittest, assuming that the hare survived its precipitous descent.

After reaching the top of Suilven, I quickly took in the panoramic view of the neighbouring peaks of Canisp and Stac Polly, then hurriedly descended as dusk started to fall. Passing deer silhouetted against the darkening sky on the adjacent hills, I arrived back at the car park just 5½ hours after I had left it, physically exhausted but spiritually refreshed. This exemplified for me the motto of the Flyfishers' Club which, translated

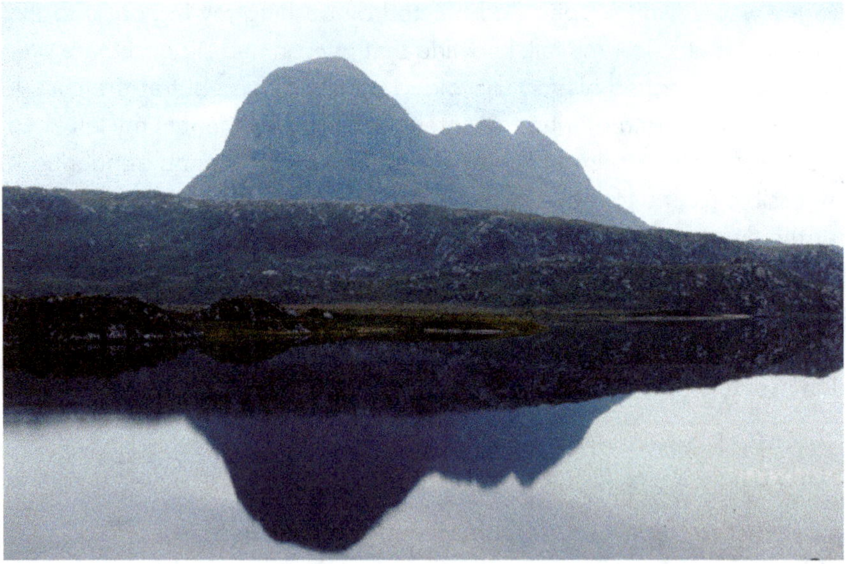

Figure 5. Suilven.

from the Latin, states "There's more to fishing than catching fish" (to which one might add "although the latter does help").

References

1. Merryweather J. Truth, lies and fish-farming. *Gamefisher* (Yearbook of Salmon & Trout Conservation UK), 2007, pp. 42–44.
2. Grimble A. *The Salmon Rivers of Scotland* (3rd edn.), 1913.

15 Hazards of Running Marathons

1994

Nineteen ninety four was a notable year for several reasons, the most important of which was the publication of 4S. It also marked the publication of a revised edition of my *Handbook of Hyperlipidaemia*,[1] which I had written in an attempt to foster greater interest in lipids and their disorders. The copyright was held by Merck, who distributed the book to GPs and physicians with an interest in the prevention and treatment of atherosclerotic cardiovascular disease and this ensured that it was widely read. More than 30,000 copies of the first edition were printed in English and it was also translated into Russian, Turkish, and Japanese. The best part of the book was the Foreword, which was written by Joe Goldstein and Mike Brown, who likened lipoprotein metabolism to the London Underground, with its capacity for shuttling passengers to and fro and its propensity to get overloaded at peak periods. They concluded that most of the problems that affect lipid transport in humans would be solved long before those that afflict the Underground. In terms of advances in knowledge of the causes and treatment of hyperlipidaemia their forecast may have been true but the practical application of that knowledge in 21st century Britain leaves much to be desired.

London Marathon

Nineteen ninety four was also the year when, in an effort to prove there was life after 60, I applied for and obtained a place to run in the London Marathon that April, conditional upon my raising £1,500 for the British Heart

Foundation. I entrusted the task of obtaining sponsors to my secretary Liz Manson, who with her charm and efficiency soon raised more than three times the sum needed. For my part, I trained by running around Wormwood Scrubs in the evenings after work, with longer runs around Richmond Park at weekends. When the day came I lined up with 25,000 other runners in Greenwich Park. It took a long time for everyone to cross the starting line but once my endorphins kicked in I found running with the crowd quite enjoyable. Fatigue started to set in after 16 miles, by Canary Wharf, and running over the cobblestones in front of the Tower of London was hard on my knees and hip-joints. Earlier in the race, I had passed a middle-aged runner who was being resuscitated unsuccessfully after sustaining a cardiac arrest (he proved to be the third fatality in the 13-year history of this event). Despite all the pasta I had consumed for several days before the race, I started to run out of glycogen along the Embankment after running about 24 miles and became hypoglycaemic. Luckily my younger son and daughter had spotted my distress and emerged from a nearby Underground station to give me a much-needed drink of carbohydrate. This restored my blood sugar and enabled me to complete the 26.2 miles in about 4½ hours, the average time for my age group. Apart from myalgia (muscle pain) in my legs I felt well after the race and dined out with friends and relatives that evening (Figure 1). I went to work as usual the next day, but in view of the persistence and severity of my myalgia I had blood taken for measurement of serum creatine kinase activity (an enzyme released from damaged muscle).[2] The results showed a total creatine kinase activity of 1,800 IU/L (normal <200 IU/L) and an MB fraction of 38 ng/mL (normal <6 ng/mL) (creatine kinase MB was regarded in those days as a specific marker of damaged heart muscle). The clinical biochemist on duty regarded my values as pathognomonic of myocardial infarction but in view of my general well-being and lack of cardiorespiratory symptoms I discounted this diagnosis. My myalgia gradually subsided, and I was jogging again within a week.

After a description of my experiences appeared in a newspaper, I received a letter from a runner who, several years previously, had been admitted to hospital after falling and sustaining concussion during a half marathon. He wrote:

> The enzyme test suggested that I had indeed had a heart attack. But I did not seem to have any of the regular

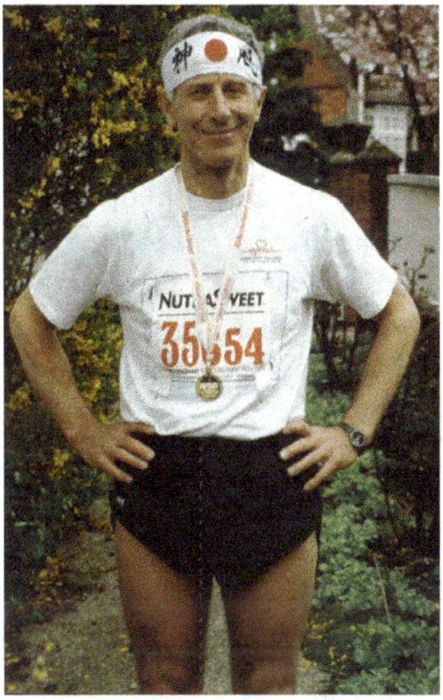

Figure 1. The author, wearing a British Heart Foundation T-shirt and kamikaze headband, after finishing the London Marathon in 1994.

> symptoms — breathlessness and the like — and I did not feel unwell. The doctor in charge told me 'marathon running is not for you, old boy.' I celebrated that by winning the National Veterans Over 55 Marathon in 2 hours 54 minutes ... only 14 months after my 'heart attack.'

He subsequently ran the London marathon in less than three hours at the age of 60!

Pseudo-myocardial infarction after a marathon is now a well-documented entity. Studies in runners in two Boston marathons showed a 15-fold increase in creatine kinase MB values 24 hours after the event.[3] Thallium scans of the heart done immediately after the marathon were normal which suggested that the increase in creatine kinase MB activity was derived from skeletal not heart muscle.[4] This was confirmed by calf muscle biopsies that showed a three-fold increase in creatine kinase MB activity during training. The conclusion was that the increase in creatine kinase MB in runners usually reflects a state of chronic muscle damage resulting from repetitive training and not a heart attack unless there is additional clinical evidence of the latter.

My myalgia soon subsided but I was taken aback to discover that I was the top fund-raising runner for the British Heart Foundation, thanks to my secretary's efforts and the generosity of my sponsors. This meant that I had won the first prize, which turned out to be a pair of BA business class return airfares to New York and a guaranteed place in the 25th Anniversary New York marathon. Running two marathons in 1 year had not been my original intention but the opportunity was too good a one to miss. The only snag was that I had damaged my knee during the summer while salmon fishing in Scotland, as described in the Chapter 14.

New York Marathon

Came November and my elder son and I disembarked from our jumbo jet at Kennedy Airport. He came to provide logistic and moral support as well as to see the sights of New York. One of the cabs we took was driven by a Ghanaian who got very excited when he heard that my son had been born in Accra. He kept stopping to communicate this piece of news to other Ghanaian cab drivers who were remarkably numerous around 42nd Street, where our hotel was.

The start of the marathon was on Staten Island, which boasts the world's longest urinal. From there the 30,000 runners ran over the two ramps of the Verrazano Narrows Bridge and then slogged along 4th Avenue through Brooklyn and into Queens before crossing the East River into Manhattan. We then ran up 1st Avenue for 4 miles (Figure 2), made a brief excursion into the Bronx, and then turned back to run down 5th Avenue. The finish was in Central Park, which was uphill all the way and a more demanding test of stamina than The Mall had been earlier in the year. It took me half an hour longer to get to the finish on my gammy knee but I did so and honour was satisfied. Sadly, I learnt afterwards that two runners had sustained fatal cardiac arrests after crossing the finishing line. That made it three deaths in the two marathons I had run and decided me against doing a third. It also stimulated me to investigate the nature and scale of the risks incurred by participants in this increasingly popular pastime.

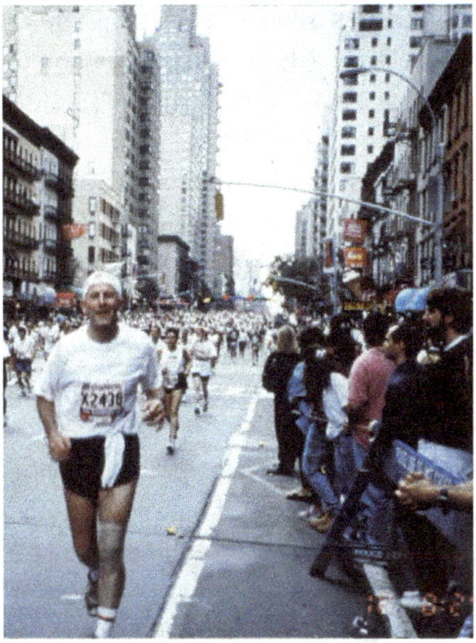

Figure 2. Slogging up 1st Avenue during the 25th New York Marathon.

Hazards of Running a Marathon

Sudden death during a marathon in younger athletes is usually due to hypertrophic cardiomyopathy (a disease of heart muscle, often inherited), but in middle-aged runners it is more often due to myocardial infarction consequent on coronary artery disease, with evidence of severe atherosclerosis at post-mortem examination. However, it is only relatively recently that sufficient data have accumulated to enable the incidence of sudden cardiac death in runners during a marathon to be reliably quantified.

The London marathon was first run in 1981 and up to 2005 there were eight sudden cardiac deaths in the 26 marathons, all in men. Five were due to coronary heart disease and three to hypertrophic cardiomyopathy.[5] An estimated total of 650,000 runners completed the course during this period, 85% of whom were male, giving an incidence of sudden cardiac death during the event of 1.25/100,000.

Most of the data on the risks of running a marathon originate from the USA where six times as many marathons are run each year as in the UK.

Furthermore, the tradition has been established there for much longer, the first Boston marathon being in 1897. A recent systematic review of sudden cardiac death in marathons analysed 7 studies published between 1996 and 2012.[6] The authors recorded a total of 106 deaths between 1975 and 2010 but accepted that there may have been some duplication of reported deaths in the various studies. The incidence of sudden cardiac death was lower in the four studies reporting 10 or more deaths (0.6–0.8 deaths/100,000 runners) than in the three studies that reported less than 10 deaths (1.2–1.9/100,000). This suggests that risk might have been over-estimated in the smaller studies or biased by demographic differences.

Analysis of the two largest US studies provided detailed information on factors influencing risk and outcomes. In one study of 3.7 million runners there were 28 deaths within 24 hours of finishing, 22 in men (0.98/100,000) and 6 in women (0.41/100,000).[7] Coronary heart disease caused 46% of all deaths and more than 90% of deaths in those aged more than 45 years. A total of 64% died after completing 20 miles and 25% died after finishing the course. In the other study, there were 59 cardiac arrests in nearly 11 million runners participating in marathons and half-marathons from 2000–2010, 42 of which were fatal.[8] The commonest cause of death in this study was hypertrophic cardiomyopathy. The authors found that the incidence of sudden cardiac death was higher in marathons than in half-marathons (0.63 versus 0.25/100,000), higher in men than women (0.62 versus 0.14/100,000) and occurred most often after 10 miles in half-marathons and after 20 miles in marathons. A strong predictor of survival after cardiac arrest was the administration of cardiopulmonary resuscitation by bystanders, especially when coronary heart disease was the underlying abnormality.

Overall the data suggest that the risk of sudden cardiac death during a marathon is very low, especially if you are female, and that it is safer to run a half-marathon than a full marathon but risky to attempt either if you have coronary heart disease or hypertrophic cardiomyopathy. Since these disorders are often covert and unsuspected, this raises the thorny question of pre-marathon screening, the case for which has both its supporters[9] and opponents.[7] Among the options being considered are a pre-participatory, 12 lead electrocardiogram to detect cardiomyopathies in younger runners and computed tomographic measurement of coronary calcification in those over the age of 50. All agree on the need for the availability of automated external defibrillators (a device that automatically diagnoses and treats arrhythmias) at marathons, especially between the 20 miles mark and the finish, where the danger of cardiac arrest is greatest. However, none of these issues detracts from the advice that advocates the cardiovascular benefits of running moderate distances on a regular basis,[10] even though this may sometimes have unintended musculoskeletal consequences. I had to give up jogging after prolapsing a lumbar intervertebral disc and now get my exercise by walking.

To conclude this chapter on a lighter but not unrelated note I will recount an episode that occurred following an arthroscopy of my damaged knee. After the procedure, I awoke from the anaesthetic feeling incredibly euphoric and looked up to see a couple of nurses in masks, both of them with Antipodean accents. In my uninhibited state of mind I asked them "Do you know what KIWI stands for?" Both replied "No": "Keenly Interested Without Intelligence" I explained. One of the nurses laughed, the other grunted and asked me "What do you do if you run over an Aussie?" I replied that I didn't know. "Reverse" she said. No prizes for guessing where she was from!

References

1. Thompson GR. *Handbook of Hyperlipidaemia*, revised edition. London: Current Science, 1994.
2. Thompson GR. Grand Rounds — Hammersmith Hospital. Hazards of running a Marathon. *BMJ* 1997;**314**:1023–5.
3. Siegel AJ, Silverman LM, Holman BL. Elevated creatine kinase MB isoenzyme levels in marathon runners. *JAMA* 1981;**246**:2049–51.
4. Siegel AJ, Silverman LM, Evans WJ. Elevated skeletal muscle creatine kinase MB isoenzyme levels in marathon runners. *JAMA* 1983;**250**:2835–7.
5. Tunstall Pedoe DS. Marathon Cardiac Deaths. The London Experience. *Sports Medicine* 2007;**37**:4–5.
6. Waite O, Smith A, Madge L, Spring H, Noret N. Sudden cardiac death in marathons: A systematic review. *Phys Sportsmed* 2016;**44**:79–84.
7. Mathews SC, Narotsky DL, Bernholt DL *et al.* Mortality among marathon runners in the United States, 2000–2009. *Am J Sports Med* 2012;**40**:1495–500.
8. Kim JH, Malhotra R, Chiampas G *et al.* Cardiac arrest during long-distance running races. *N Eng J Med* 2012;**366**:130–40.

9. Corrado D, Pelliccia A, Bjornstad HH *et al.* Cardiovascular pre-participation screening of young competitive athletes for prevention of sudden death: Proposal for a common European protocol: Consensus statement of the Study Group of Sport Cardiology of the Working Group of Cardiac Rehabilitation and Exercise Physiology and the Working Group of Myocardial and Pericardial Diseases of the European Society of Cardiology. *Eur Heart J* 2005;**26**:516–24.
10. Pate RR, Pratt M, Blair SN *et al.* Physical activity and public health. A recommendation from the Centers for Disease Control and Prevention and the American College of Sports Medicine. *JAMA* 1995;**273**:402–7.

16 Exuma

The Bahamas Connection

Exuma — the word conjures up memories of blissful family holidays and one of the most exciting fishing experiences of my life. It is the collective name for the islands of Great and Little Exuma, which are linked by a short bridge, and is the largest and most southerly of the Exuma Cays, a chain of islands in the Bahamas stretching south east from Nassau for over 100 miles.

My love affair with Exuma arose from the generosity of an American patient of mine who worked in London. He had heterozygous FH and progressive coronary disease, both of which were very difficult to treat. This was in the pre-statin era so we decided to try to get his cholesterol as low as possible by asking one of our surgeons to perform an ileal bypass operation. In this procedure, the intestinal contents bypass the ileum (the terminal part of the small intestine where bile acids are reabsorbed). Bile acids are synthesised from cholesterol and their increased loss from the body following this procedure resulted in a compensatory increase in the conversion of cholesterol into bile acids and a dramatic lowering of the patient's cholesterol. Afterwards, with typical American generosity he very kindly offered to lend me his house in Exuma for a couple of weeks. He and his wife used it as a holiday home in those days but intended to retire there permanently after he had wound up his publishing business in London.

George Town

My wife, younger daughter, and I first landed in Exuma in November 1979 on a Bahamas Air flight from Miami. As we touched down on the tiny airstrip at George Town, the administrative capital, we were greeted by the sobering sight of a wrecked plane in the undergrowth bordering the runway. The airport terminal consisted of a large hut with a sign on the front which read "250th Anniversary of Parliament," referring to the establishment of the first General Assembly of the Bahamas in 1729. A smaller hut nearby labelled "Kermit's" turned out to be a bar. Two large taxis, probably the only ones on the island, were parked in the shade of some nearby trees. After a perfunctory customs and immigration check I hired one of the taxis to take my wife, younger daughter aged 2, and myself to Hi-Ho, the house that had been lent to us by our American friends.

The house was built on a small hill on the windward side of the island within sight of the sea and was cooled in the evenings by a gentle breeze. It was well equipped and comfortable but there was one snag when we arrived — no water. The power station in George Town had burnt down a couple of weeks previously and the electricity supply for the entire town was provided by an emergency generator on a rota basis. The water supply to Hi-Ho was normally pumped up from a well by an electric pump but, without electricity, the pump had lost its prime. Luckily our neighbour helped us to re-prime it by running a hosepipe from his water tank to our pump and filling the pipe from the well by gravity. Thanks to him we could thenceforth draw water from the well whenever the power came on.

We rented a Mini-Moke and explored the island both north and south of George Town by driving along the King's Highway, a pot-holed tarmac road which ran the length of Exuma. The island exuded old fashioned charm and its friendly inhabitants assumed you would stop and give them a lift if you were going in their direction, cars being a scarce commodity. The beaches were long stretches of white sand, uncontaminated in those days by the needles discarded by drug addicts in later years (Figure 1). Further evidence of the drug problem in the 1980s and 1990s was the wreck on one of the beaches of a drug runner's plane that ran out of fuel while *en route* from South America. These planes used to drop boxes containing illegal narcotics into the sea off the US coast to be collected by drug dealers using motorboats, an activity described by Bahamians as "Square Grouper" fishing. Exuma was on the flight path to Florida and the US Drug Enforcement Agency positioned a radar balloon in the sky above

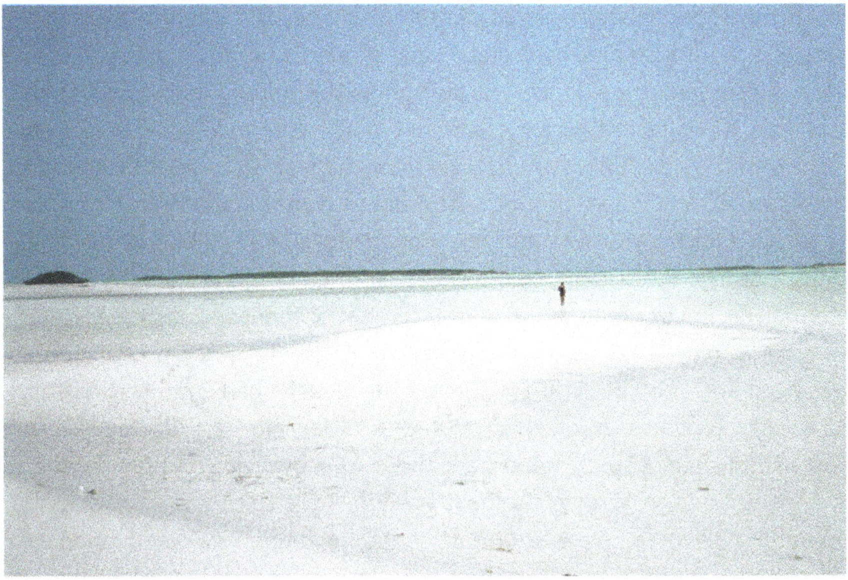

Figure 1. Coco Plum Beach, Exuma.

George Town to detect and track unauthorised aircraft and alert the US Coastguard accordingly.

During that first visit I hired a guide to take me out for a day's bone-fishing, a novel experience for me. We set off in his boat from Moss Town and once we got to the bonefish flats my guide gave me a spinning rod to cast a hook baited with shrimp or crab meat into "mud," patches of muddy water created by a school of bonefish when bottom feeding. Casting blind into "mud" nearly always caught a bonefish, most of them weighing 2 or 3 lb. They fought well but it was an unsatisfying method of catching them. Getting them to take a fly is much harder but far more exciting, as I discovered on subsequent visits when I brought a fly rod with me.

The Rolle Dynasty

Exuma has an interesting history. The Bahamas were first colonised by Britain in 1629, in the reign of Charles 1. The earliest settlement was on the island of Eleuthera but Nassau soon became the main focus of colonial activity. Most of the settlers on Exuma were British Loyalists, who had migrated there from Georgia and South Carolina in the 1780s when their land, property, and businesses were confiscated after Britain lost the American War of Independence. In pre-Loyalist times the population of Exuma was less than 40 white settlers and black slaves all told. However, it was greatly augmented by the influx of Loyalists after the war who, attracted by land grants from the Crown, brought their slaves with them with the intention of establishing cotton plantations similar to those they had left behind. Unfortunately, the soil on Exuma was of such poor quality that the cotton plantations never really prospered and most of them soon petered out.

One name that constantly crops up in Exuma is Rolle. Denys Rolle was born and bred in Devon and was a Member of Parliament. An idealist he sought and was granted 20,000 acres of land in East Florida in 1767 and established a small settlement there for down and outs he brought over from London. During the next few years the settlement grew in size up until 1783 when, in the aftermath of the Revolutionary War, Florida was returned to Spain. In compensation for the consequent loss of his land in Florida the Crown granted Rolle large tracts of land in Exuma, where he transported his slaves, livestock, and possessions in a vessel called the "Peace & Plenty," the name subsequently adopted by the main hotel and night spot in George Town (Figure 2). Denys Rolle died in 1797 and his land and slaves were inherited by his son, Lord John Rolle. The latter never lived in Exuma but many of his 325 slaves took his name when Britain abolished slavery in 1834. It was subsequently perpetuated in two towns, Rolle Town and Rolleville, and now half the population of Exuma seems to be named Rolle: Kermit's bar was owned by Kermit Rolle, one of the taxi drivers was Willie Rolle, and the best bonefish guides on the island were Will and Sam Rolle, of whom more anon.

My family and I returned to Exuma on numerous occasions between 1983 and 1993, usually in late July and early August, when only mad dogs and Englishmen brave the midday sun. We would fly from London to Miami, spend the afternoon and night in a cheap motel near the airport (it had a pool and served very cold beer) and then catch an early morning flight to George Town. The plane was usually a twin engine Cessna which could just about accommodate us all. Before we boarded the pilot would say "Well, who's going to be co-pilot today?" a task usually performed by my doctor son-in-law. The view from the plane of the sea, sapphire blue

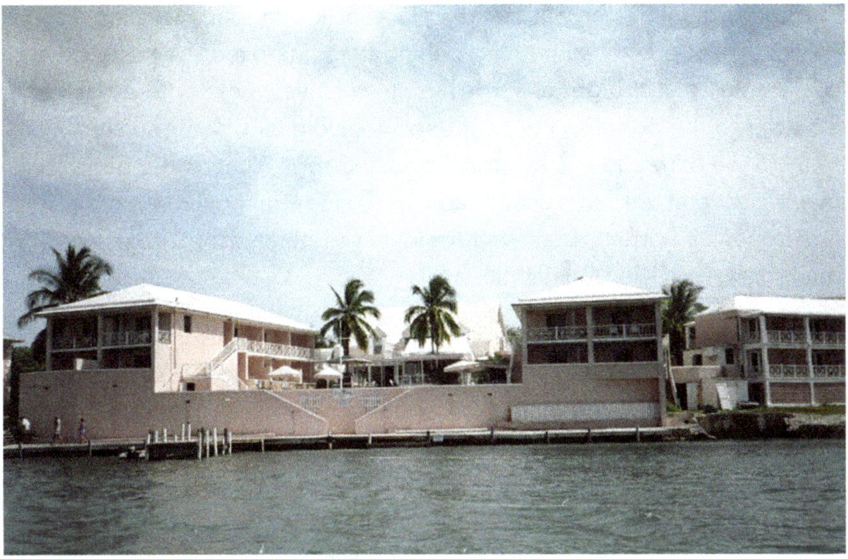

Figure 2. The Peace and Plenty Hotel, Exuma.

where the water was deep and turquoise green where it was shallow, and of the white islands 8,000 feet below us was spectacular.

Peace and Plenty

Our American friend and his wife were now living in Hi-Ho so we rented a house nearby, overlooking the sea. On Friday nights we'd join them for the dance at the Peace and Plenty, the highlight of the social week in George Town in the summer, with music provided by the Goombay Band led by a talented local singer, George Wylie. His Bahamian songs had catchy melodies but rather risqué lyrics, such as "Who put the pepper in the Vaseline?" The combination of his soothing voice and cool Kalik beer while sitting out under the stars at the Peace and Plenty was the perfect ending to a day spent wading the bonefish flats in the blazing sunshine.

We used to rent a Boston Whaler with an outboard engine from the local boatyard, one of the few non-Rolle businesses in George Town, in which we explored Elizabeth Harbour and went water skiing. One year the Bahamian owner, a keen fisherman, was seriously injured in a freak accident which occurred while he was standing in a shallow lagoon watching a shoal of bonefish. Suddenly something behind them spooked the bonefish and they accelerated straight towards him. Instinctively he stepped back and as he did so the bonefish turned steeply to avoid him. Their pursuer, however, a large barracuda came straight on and took a chunk out of his foot, severing several tendons, presumably mistaking the movement of his foot for a bonefish. Barracudas have formidable teeth and they, together with small sharks, are the bonefish's main predators.

Shark Channel

Speaking of sharks recalls the occasion when my American friend and I decided to visit a small island situated on the bonefish flats on the leeward side of the island, not far from the airport. To get there involved driving along a series of deserted roads with impressive names like Zebrafish Drive. These roads were flanked by vacant concrete housing plots, now overgrown by vegetation, which had originally been placed there and sold by a developer but had never been built upon. Just off one of these roads was a path through the undergrowth that led to the sea and we used it to carry an inflatable rubber dinghy down to the water's edge. After inflating the dinghy we launched it and started paddling towards the island across a stretch of water known as the Shark Channel. Half way across we suddenly saw two large black dorsal fins bearing down upon us. Instantly our leisurely progress was transformed into a frantic burst of paddling as we strove to get to the island before the sharks got to us, which we just managed. Shark attacks are said to be rare in the Bahamas but we didn't intend to put this notion to the test.

The island had some trees on it where a pair of ospreys nested each year. Like barracuda and sharks, ospreys are bonefish predators and whenever their shadow fell across a shoal of bonefish in shallow water the latter would erupt with a loud splash as the fish took evasive action *en masse*. I later discovered that it was quite easy to wade across the Shark Channel at low tide without the need for a boat and thereby gain access to a vast area of bonefish flats. I used to wade these flats in shorts and a T-shirt in warm, translucent water on firm white sand all day long. However, the reflection off the surface of the sea of the sun's vertical rays was a health hazard and my legs got badly sunburned before I got wise and learned to wear long trousers on my first few days out on the flats. Another hazard was stingrays, which could be avoided by shuffling over the sandy bottom in plimsolls, thereby pushing rays out of the way instead of treading on them.

The foremost requirement of flyfishing for bonefish is being able to spot them. This is not easy, even with the help of very dark Polaroids — bonefish are known as the "grey ghosts of the flats" because they blend in so well with their surroundings. Having learned how to spot them the next challenge is to cast a weighted fly accurately in front of them, often into a strong sea breeze, and to do so without creating too much of a splash. One then strips the line in to get the fly to mimic the movement of a crustacean on the sea bed. If a bonefish sees the fly and takes it, all Hell then breaks loose as it rips off 10 yards of line per second — it's like being attached to Usain Bolt. I had a reel disintegrate during one such run and on another occasion got my thumb burnt by the friction of the departing line.

This form of fishing was free and great fun but the fish were seldom very large. Also if the day's end coincided with high tide I then had the slightly fraught task of wading back across the Shark Channel, with water up to my chin and my fishing rod held in both hands above my head, feeling distinctly vulnerable. Once the crossing had been safely achieved there was just the small task of getting back to the car without being bitten to death by mosquitoes and "no see ums" (sand flies).

A Big Bonefish

To have the chance of catching a big bonefish necessitated hiring a good guide at a cost of $200 a day. The best guide in Exuma was Will Rolle, who lived in Rolle Town and knew all there was to know about bonefish (Figure 3). He was a tall, sparely built man with a quiet voice and a very black skin. I fished with him on several occasions over the years and he took me to some excellent spots in his boat. We would meet early in the morning at the beach near the now disused old airport, which had been superseded by a newer, bigger one. Will had his outboard engine going flat out *en route* to our destination for the day, which often involved travelling a considerable distance in his flat-bottomed boat, bouncing along on top of the water as we went. Once we neared the target area Will would cut

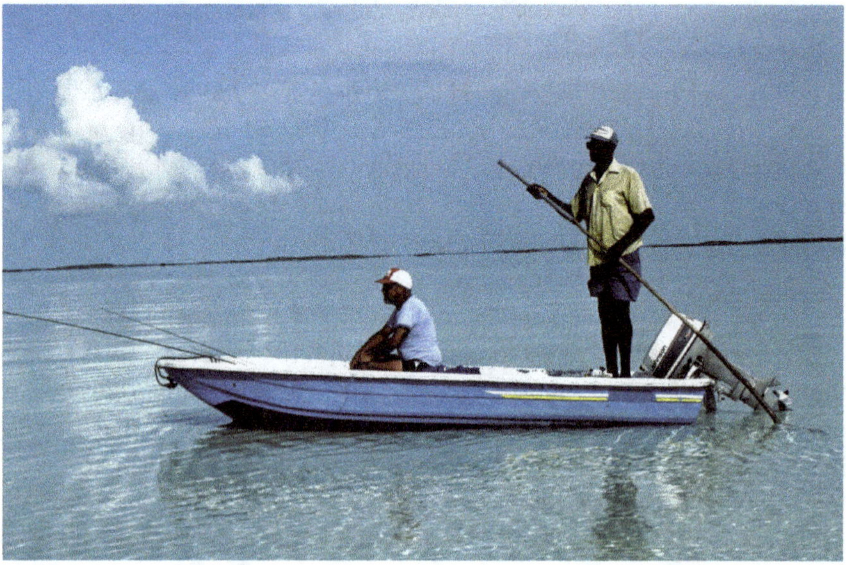

Figure 3. Will Rolle and client searching for bonefish, Exuma.

the engine and switch to poling the boat like a punt. He could spot fish long before I did and would quietly specify their whereabouts in clockwise terms. About the only occasion when it is easy to spot bonefish is if they are tailing in shallow water, when their tails flash in the sun like sails in a regatta.

My most successful and memorable bonefishing exploit was in the summer of 1992, when Will took me and my younger daughter, then aged 14, out to a distant cay. Once there Will suggested that I should get out of the boat and start wading over a wide, white sandy flat bordered by mangroves, a favourite haunt of bonefish. They would swim into the mangroves with the incoming tide in search of crustaceans and then drift out when the tide turned. However, if a hooked bonefish went into the mangroves the line usually got wrapped around their roots and the fish nearly always got off.

On this occasion I was wading out in the open, in water 2–3 feet deep, when I spotted a very large bonefish about 30 yards ahead of me, accompanied by two much smaller outriders. All three bonefish were coming slowly in my direction, with the smaller ones several yards in front of and to either side of the big one. This meant that I had to cast my fly so that it fell between and behind the two small bonefish, without either attracting or spooking them, and in front of but not too close to the big one. I realised that I had only one chance to achieve this objective but despite the fact that I was using a 10½ feet #7 weight rod, I managed to cast the fly, a Lead Eye Charlie, so that it landed more or less where I intended. As the big fish slowly came nearer, probing the seabed with its nose, I started to strip the line in so as to make the fly hop towards me along the sand. As soon as it saw the fly move the big fish sped forward and grabbed it. I struck hard and the reel screamed as the bonefish shot off, intermittently bouncing along the surface of the water as it went. After taking 100 yards or so of line and backing, the fish then paused for breath, metaphorically speaking, while I desperately attempted to reel in the line. After a further series of explosive runs, each a little shorter than the previous one, the fish began to tire and I was able to recover the backing and most of my line. As it swam around me in ever decreasing circles I started worrying that by slowing the fish down I would make it vulnerable to attack by a marauding barracuda or small shark, leaving nothing but the fish's head on the end of my line. However, all's well that ends well, and Will duly netted the bonefish and my daughter took a photo of its delighted captor. It weighed 9½ lb and Will took it home to Rolle Town for supper (not recommended). And so ended a red letter day in the life of this very lucky fisherman.

Three days later, our holiday over, we all climbed into a Cessna and took off for Miami. *En route* we saw the huge mass of menacing black clouds in the distance that denoted Hurricane Andrew heading towards South Florida, having battered Eleuthera with 170 mph winds. Fortunately, we got to Miami before it did and were lucky to catch the last flight out to London amid chaotic scenes that prefaced the closure of the airport for several days.

17 Russia

Perestroika

The installation of Mikhail Gorbachev as General Secretary of the Communist Party of the Soviet Union in 1985 marked the beginning of the end of the Cold War and the eventual dissolution of the Soviet Union. In 1989, Communist governments started collapsing like dominos, initially in Poland, then Hungary and Czechoslovakia, soon followed by the fall of the Berlin Wall and the East German government. The process was completed in 1991 when Boris Yeltsin led the counter-revolution in Russia that resulted in the resignation of President Gorbachev and the dissolution of the USSR. Yeltsin became President of the Russian Federation but there followed 8 years of political unrest, economic crisis, and social anarchy, culminating in his resignation at the end of 1999.

Moscow and Leningrad

It was during this time of change that I was invited to Russia (or USSR as it was then) initially in May and then again in November 1988 to lecture at the Cardiology Research Centre and other venues. My hosts put me up in the unpronounceable Mezhdunarodnaya Hotel which overlooks the Moskva River. They took me to see the Kremlin, with its impressive buildings, towers, and cathedrals and of course Red Square with its Disneyesque St. Basil's Cathedral (Figure 1). In front of the latter is the circular Lobnoye Mesto, from where Ivan the Terrible addressed his subjects, or in some accounts executed them, and in the distance Lenin's Tomb which looks across Red Square towards the huge Gum store that had virtually nothing

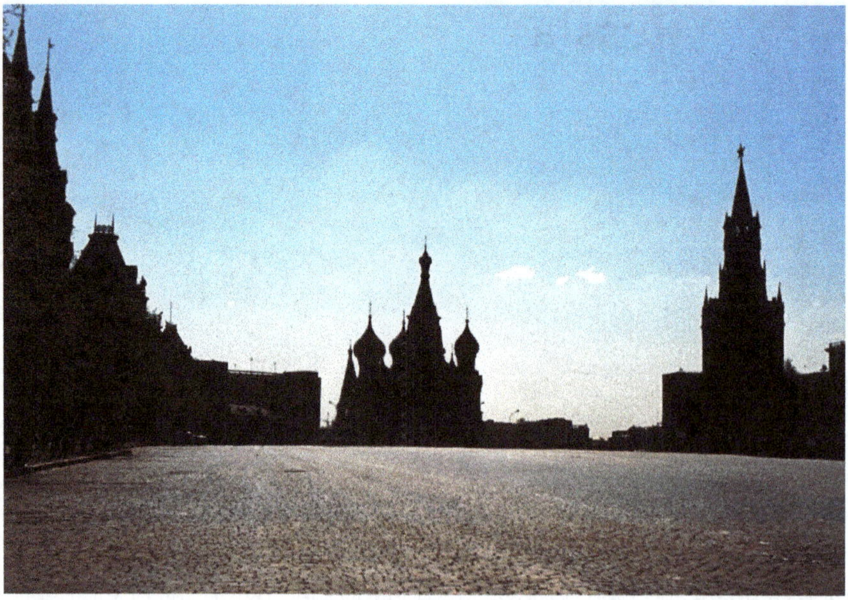

Figure 1. Red Square, Moscow, with St. Basil's Cathedral and the Spasskaya Tower in silhouette.

in it to buy. Outside were a group of old soldiers, laden with medals, who had come to Moscow for the May Day parade. The only sign of Western influence was a vending machine labelled COKN (Coke). We travelled from place to place in a van with drawn curtains but I never discovered whether this was to prevent me from seeing or being seen.

I returned in December the following year, this time accompanied by my wife, to lecture in snowbound Moscow and we then took the train to Leningrad (now St. Petersburg), where it was so cold that the Neva River was frozen over. My wife had wisely brought her racoon fur coat and hat with her, which she'd acquired during our stay in Montreal, and I quickly bought myself a fur hat with ear flaps. We, *de rigueur*, visited L'Hermitage Museum and Palace Square, where the Bolsheviks sacked the adjacent Winter Palace in 1917. On Sunday we went to a large Russian Orthodox church that was packed with local worshippers and stood throughout the 2-hour service, fascinated by the elaborate ceremonial of the priests and transfixed by the superb singing of the choir.

The Kola Peninsula

My next visit to Russia was at the beginning of the new Millennium and for a completely different reason. The year 2000 had started with a bang, or rather a multitude of bangs as London welcomed the 21st century with a dazzling fireworks display and New Year's Eve parties galore. What better way to celebrate it I thought, after sobering up, than with a fishing trip to the Kola Peninsula in Russia. Roxton Bailey Robinson was offering an experimental end of season week at $3,900 per rod, including accommodation, food, drink, and helicopter flights. The obvious companion for this venture was Tim Haskins, a friend from Thomas's days and a fanatical salmon fisherman. It didn't take long to persuade him that it was too good an opportunity to miss — it never did take long if he thought there was a chance of catching a salmon.

Friday, September 8th, started early with an 8 am flight to Edinburgh, where I had a lecture to give that morning. This accomplished I flew back to Heathrow, took a taxi home to Chiswick to meet Tim, picked up my fishing gear and returned to Heathrow just in time to catch the 6 pm Finnair flight to Helsinki. After a brief overnight stay in a Holiday Inn we made our way to the airport early the next morning with our bags and rods, mine a double-handed 15-feet Sage in its K.I.S. (Keep It Safe) case. I had bought the rod brand new a month or two earlier, following an unforgettable Spey casting lesson by a well-known and flamboyant instructor on a weed infested pond. He emphasised the timing of the various manoeuvres with exhortations along the lines of "wait for it, wait for it — *now*, as the actress said to the bishop!" Half way through the lesson he put me on the spot and told me that I needed to decide there and then whether or not to buy the rod. Happily I decided to do so and I have greatly enjoyed using it ever since.

Suitably equipped with rods, Simms waders, and boots and a wading staff (vital), and armed with a selection of flies from Farlow's, I embarked with Tim on our trip to the Arctic Circle. The atmosphere in Helsinki Airport on these occasions and details of the subsequent journey have been inimitably captured by Charles Gaines in his article "Paradise is a river in Russia" and in his book *Waters Far and Near.*[1] He describes the scene in the departure hall at crack of dawn where groups of middle-aged men queue up to check in for the Finnair flight to Murmansk, each group betraying its nationality by the facial expressions and sartorial characteristics of its members. These included Americans, Frenchmen, Spaniards, and Britons, among whom I featured as "an English doctor with a bottle of single malt Scotch peeking out of his backpack." There was also a solitary Japanese fisherman, who turned out to be the international sales manager for Daiwa, with whom Charles Gaines had a staccato question and answer session along the following lines: "Where you go in Russia?" asked the Japanese salesman "Kharlovka, Rynda and East Litza" said Charles — "and you?" "Umba" he replied, "then Kharlovka and Rynda. You fish in salt water? This year I been to Cuba, Solomon Islands, Belize, Guam." When asked whether he did anything other than fish he thought for a moment and then replied "Travel to get there!"

Charles Gaines went on to describe our journey from Murmansk in an old MI-8 helicopter with nothing but the desolate tundra below us and the crash of a smaller helicopter the previous year, when a group of fishermen based in another camp were stranded on a river bank for 12 hours without medical assistance. Their repeated Mayday calls went unanswered, despite the fact that one of the fishermen on board had sustained a pneumothorax (a collapsed lung) and was in a precarious state. When they failed to return for supper their fishing lodge on the Varzina sent out a rescue party and thankfully found them in time.

The Kola is a 40,000 square miles peninsula that protrudes into the Arctic Circle and is bordered on the north by the Barents Sea and by the White Sea on the east. It is inhabited mainly by reindeer and nomadic Samii and is invaded each summer by salmon fishermen attracted by its reputation for providing what is arguably the best salmon fishing in the world. Much of this is due to an Englishman called Peter Power and it was to the fishing camps he owned that we were bound. Our first stop was the camp on the Rynda, where some of us disembarked, while the remainder journeyed on to the camp on the Kharlovka. The third river, the East Litza, has only a small tent camp manned by a resident river warden.

Now in his 70s, Peter Power is a larger than life character in several respects, both in physique and personality — he is well over 6 feet tall and has a matching ego — and in terms of his achievements. He made a fortune from building up and then selling a company which manufactured plastic strapping for wrapping bundles of newspapers. With too much money to burn and too much spare time he soon became an alcoholic. He eventually came to realise that he had to give up drinking before it killed him and managed to do so successfully. This left him free to pursue in no uncertain manner his passion for salmon fishing. But more importantly he made it possible for others to share in his passion by leasing the fishing rights to three of the best rivers in the Kola Peninsula. During the 2002 season almost 3,500 salmon were caught and released by paying guests like Tim and myself. These averaged 14 lb with 50 fish weighing more than 30 lb each and 5 more than 40 lb. As Charles Gaines puts it, in terms of Atlantic salmon fishing that is "Best in Show."

His account recaptures perfectly the atmosphere of setting out for a week's fishing in the Kola Peninsula, including the Soviet-style mandatory half hour that it took each of us to pass the scrutiny of grim-faced Russian immigration and customs officials at Murmansk before we were allowed to board our helicopter. One year we were fog bound there for the night, an experience I never wish to repeat. My hotel room door was nearly smashed open at midnight by a drunken Russian who had mistaken my room for his, where his girlfriend was waiting for him. But once we were *en route* to the Rynda and Kharlovka fishing camps the atmosphere changed to one of excitement and the Russians who accompanied us and who staffed the camps became cheerful and friendly, helpful, and sober — they were not allowed to drink alcohol in camp. But that didn't stop us from doing so, to celebrate our successes on the river or to console ourselves for our losses and the malt whisky I had bought at Heathrow soon disappeared.

There would be plenty of opportunities to experience both these emotions during the week ahead and we faced it with unbridled optimism. This contrasted with the increasing pessimism that I felt about fishing in Scotland in those days, especially on the west coast, where the proliferation of fish farms has led to ever decreasing runs of salmon and especially sea trout. Sadly, the negative effects of fish farms counteract the benefits that have resulted from the late Orri Vigfusson's hugely successful efforts to reduce commercial fishing for salmon at sea and the netting of salmon at the mouths of rivers. An unwelcome example of the Third Law of Physics in operation.

In 1998, Peter Power leased from the Russian authorities 20 million acres of the Kola Peninsula and the fishing rights to the three Northern

Rivers and bought the camps on the Rynda and Kharlovka rivers. One of his first tasks was to eliminate the poaching of fish that was rife at the time. It may be apocryphal but the story goes that there was a Russian radar station at the mouth of the Kharlovka, put there during the Cold War era to give early warning of intercontinental ballistic missiles launched by the West. After the collapse of the Soviet Union the unit had been more or less forgotten by the military and the soldiers based there were getting increasingly short of supplies of food and fuel. Peter Power offered to provide both these necessities in exchange for anti-poaching patrols by armed soldiers in helicopters. He soon replaced them with civilian river wardens and the introduction of such measures on the three rivers had a dramatic effect on poaching. Their adoption, together with a mandatory catch and release policy, has resulted in a steady increase every year in the number of salmon returning to spawn. Quite an achievement in this day and age!

Salmon Fishing on the Three Rivers

On my first visit to the Kola in 2000, the Kharlovka camp had already closed for the season so Tim and I stayed at the Rynda camp, which Peter Power usually reserved for his close friends. Peter was very hospitable and we used to chat with him in the evenings over a drink, in his case a soft one. We fished mainly on the Rynda but went over to the Kharlovka by helicopter a couple of times during the week.

We were there in September, which is when the Osenka (icefish) spawn, having entered the river the previous winter and spent it under the ice. Despite having been in fresh water for a year these fish were fatter than standard salmon but silver grey in colour rather than the mint silver of fresh run fish. Tim went out one afternoon in a boat on the Home pool of the Rynda and caught a 25 lb Osenka. My best fish that year was a modest 15 pounder on the Kharlovka but it was the largest salmon I had caught up till then and it whetted my appetite for bigger ones.

Since it was September, the days were getting shorter and the nights longer and colder. On clear nights we were treated to a superb display of the Northern Lights, a shimmering curtain of green fluorescence that waxed and waned low down in the starry sky. Already there was ice on the duck boards in the mornings and soon the Arctic winter would set in and encase the camp, river, and surrounding tundra in a white blanket of snow and ice until the following May. It was time for us to head back home.

I returned to the Kola annually for the next 4 years but on my own. Tim's knees were too unstable for him to wade in comfort and safety and none of my other fishing acquaintances were keen to accompany me, either because they were too busy or because of the considerable expense involved. Fishing rotas were arranged on the basis of two fishermen per guide so I had to take pot luck when I got there as to who I fished with. Often I was on my own but sometimes the fishing manager, a superb fisherman, partnered me and gave me much needed advice on how to improve my Spey casting.

Apart from that first visit to the Rynda, I stayed at the Kharlovka camp on all my subsequent trips between 2001 and 2004. During that period there was a steady improvement in the standard of comfort provided by the wooden huts in which we fishermen were accommodated and nowadays each hut has its own *en suite* facilities. The food was excellent, shipped in from elsewhere by helicopter but cooked by Russian chefs in the camp kitchen. Breakfast and supper were taken in the communal dining room where fishermen and guides ate together, while lunch was provided on the river bank by one's guide. It always included soup heated up on a primus stove, come rain or shine. Hot soup was extremely welcome during the second week in June 2003, when the river banks were still covered in snow and lumps of ice floated past while I waded in numbingly cold water. I failed to catch anything that week except a kelt (fish that has recently spawned). In complete contrast, hot soup was totally inappropriate at the end of July the following year when, under a blazing sun, I had to cover my face and neck with a net to prevent the voracious Russian mosquitoes from eating me alive.

The large Home Pool at the Kharlovka was within easy walking distance of the camp and always full of fish. There was always enough light in mid-summer to fish there 24 hours a day but the wading was treacherous because of the uneven height of the boulders and strength of the current. I would often fish there late on the final night of the week on the "Last Chance Saloon" principle and inevitably I always fell in. This meant having to pack wet boots and sodden clothes in my luggage for the return journey the next day. Not unexpectedly, this failed to evoke much sympathy when I got home to London.

If one was due to fish the East Litza, this entailed a hectic rush in the morning in order to be ready for the punctual departure of the small helicopter assigned to take us there, small that is in comparison with the ex-Afghan War MI-8 that brought us from Murmansk. We soon learned how to crouch down under the rotating blades and how to get ourselves and all our fishing gear in and out of the chopper in a hurry, *M*A*S*H*-style. We also learned the need to be punctual at the rendezvous for the return trip if one was to avoid spending the night there. Having a fish on was not an acceptable excuse for lateness. That said there is a Tent Camp on the Litza where a helicopter is parked overnight and where one can stay as a guest of Vassily, the rugged resident guardian who uses a Kalashnikov to kill bears and frighten poachers, although just the sight of him should achieve the latter objective.

Like many others who have fished the Three Rivers the Litza is my favourite, partly because of its beauty, epitomised by the magnificent Litza Falls Pool (Figure 2), above which no salmon can go, and partly because of the size of its fish. The latter feature was exemplified by Adrian Latimer in his book *Paradise Found*[2] where he describes in graphic detail how he caught a huge cock salmon in Flat Stone Pool, not far below the Litza Falls. This fish had an estimated weight of 46½ lb and as he says in the book, it was a fish of several lifetimes.

In fishing terms, my most productive trips were the first week in July 2001 and the third week in June 2002. On the first of these occasions my guide was Velodya, who spoke quite good English. We went over to the Litza one day when it rained steadily, rather like Scotland on a summer's day. After a considerable amount of walking and scrambling we eventually came to what Velodya called Secret Place, a small pool situated at the end of a fast run under a cliff that formed the opposite bank. I cast my fly, a green Temple Dog, into the run and as it went into the deeper water there was a huge boil beside it but the line remained slack. "Change fly" said Velodya. I duly obliged by putting on a red Temple Dog and cast it out as before. The boil was repeated but this time the line went taut and Velodya eventually netted a beautiful, bright silver salmon weighing 22 lb, which was soon followed by its 16 lb younger cousin (Figure 2).

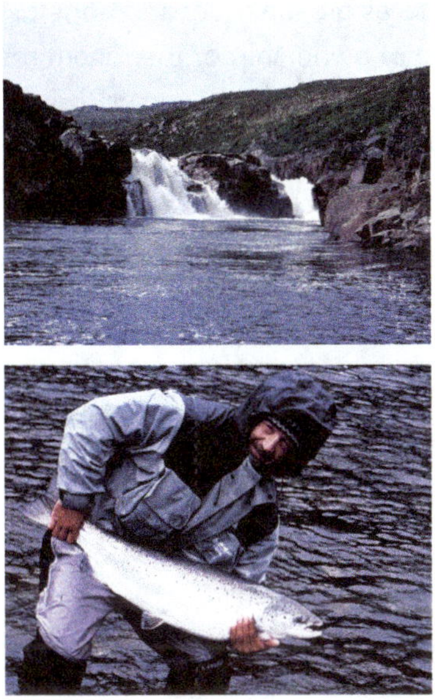

Figure 2. East Litza Falls (upper image) and fresh-run 22 lb salmon about to be returned to the river (lower image).

I did even better the following year when my guide was Oleg, who spoke no English. We communicated in sign language and he helped me to catch 10 fish during the week, averaging 13 lb, the largest again being 22 lb, which I caught in Lower Tent Pool on the Litza. Landing this salmon involved some hair-raising rock hopping by Oleg. I also caught a 19 lb fish just below the Kharlovka Falls Pool, which it took me 1½ hours to prize off the bottom of the river. I was standing on a ledge of rock with the fish directly below me in deep water and I could only apply upwards but not sideways strain. I lost six fish that week, some of them very large and quite unstoppable despite 20 lb breaking strain nylon. However, to put my modest achievements into their proper perspective, Peter Power brought his lifetime tally of salmon weighing 30 lb or more to five before the season ended! I have yet to catch a single one of that size.

Peter Power renamed his Northern Rivers (Three Rivers) venture The Atlantic Salmon Reserve in 2003, which has a strongly conservation-orientated mandate binding on all future owners, and then sold it to the Russian-owned Kharlovka Company in 2011. The demand for fishing reservations seems to be as great as ever and hopefully will not be adversely affected by the change of ownership or the recent resurgence of Cold War attitudes in Russia. To fish the Three Rivers is the experience of a lifetime for those who enjoy both fishing for salmon and the fringe benefits that go with it. Where else in the world would you have an audience, as I once did, of a covey of astonishingly tame ptarmigan watching you fish while sunning themselves after their meal of cloud berries pecked from the tundra? The latter may look like a barren wasteland, which of course it is for most of the year, and scenically it is far less attractive than the Scottish highlands. But this is offset by the magnificence of the rivers that rush through it on their way down to the Barents Sea and by the size, strength, and number of salmon that run up them. The pleasure of fishing those rivers will remain with me long after I've forgotten the pain of how much it cost me to do so.

References

1. Gaines C. *Waters Far and Near.* Guilford, USA: Lyons Press, 2015.
2. Latimer A. *Paradise Found.* Adrian Latimer, 2002.

18 Retirement

Reorganisation

In 1997, the Royal Postgraduate Medical School ceased to exist as such and was subsumed into the Faculty of Medicine of Imperial College London. Inevitably, this resulted in a loss of the sense of uniqueness and independence that had characterised the institution. The Department of Medicine was replaced by the Division of Medicine, a vertical structure that included staff working in other institutions within Imperial College such as the undergraduate medical schools of St. Mary's and Charing Cross and Westminster. Unfortunately, all were on separate sites so that the advantages of closer physical contacts with more colleagues was hypothetical. The increasing specialisation of Medicine has made people reluctant to discuss topics outside their area of expertise, a tendency that will undoubtedly become more marked with the increasing domination of molecular biology and genetics. In the long run this could presage the demise of clinical research at the Hammersmith, which would be sad. Although spoken more than 80 years ago in his Harveian Oration on "Clinical Science," the words of the great Welsh cardiologist Sir Thomas Lewis are as relevant now as they were then: "Knowledge that is applied usefully to the health of mankind will almost always come by a series of steps, the first of which is the recognition of the human need, the last of which is the application of a test directly to the human problem. It is therefore in the nature of things, however many steps may intervene, that the first and last shall be clinical."[1]

In 2019, the Faculty of Medicine was reorganised yet again, a process that included eliminating the Department or Division of Medicine altogether and dividing the Faculty into eight academic departments including four new ones, namely Infectious Disease; Immunology and Inflammation; Brain Sciences; and Metabolism, Digestion and Reproduction — the last of these departments combines an extraordinary juxtaposition of disciplines. Hopefully, these changes will not sound the death knell for the Medical Staff Round at the Hammersmith, where generations of clinicians have learnt how to present complex cases to a critical audience with a wide range of interests.

Retirement

By the autumn of 1998, I had reached the mandatory retirement age for MRC clinical staff of 65. This was too early for my liking — unnecessarily so I thought, it was not as if I was a cardiac surgeon needing precise eye–hand coordination for my work. My value, such as it was, lay in my experience of diagnosing and of managing different forms of hyperlipidaemia over many years, knowledge that does not fade with age and which was in short supply in Britain at that time. However, this was still in the ageism era so I reluctantly said *au revoir* to my MRC and Imperial College colleagues and erstwhile research fellows, who generously organised a Festschrift and dinner for me at the Hammersmith. I said goodbye to my patients in the Lipid Clinic and handed over their care to my successor, Rossi Naoumova. I also bade a sad farewell to my secretary so it soon became obvious that my most urgent task was to learn how to use a computer, send emails, and make my own Powerpoint slides.

The title of Professor of Clinical Lipidology had been conferred on me by the Royal Postgraduate Medical School in 1996 and after my retirement Imperial College awarded me Emeritus status. I maintained an active interest in lipids by becoming the medical advisor to McNeil Nutritionals and helped them launch their cholesterol-lowering spread Benecol. The active constituent is plant stanol ester, which works by interfering with the absorption of cholesterol from the small intestine, and I took the opportunity to supervise a South African research fellow's PhD on this topic. I also kept my clinical hand in by seeing private patients at the Cromwell Hospital in South Kensington until I reached the age when medical insurers would no longer reimburse my consultation fees. Nowadays, my only remaining clinical contact is attending the audit session that follows the weekly Lipid

Clinic at Hammersmith Hospital, where my colleagues discuss their patients and I then review the latest publications on lipids and CVD. Keeping up to date with the literature used to necessitate regular visits to the Wellcome Library at the Hammersmith but is achievable nowadays with a click of the mouse on my laptop, thanks to search programmes such as Zetoc Alert and the ability to get access to millions of citations via the US National Library of Medicine's PubMed.

Publications

I continued to publish scientific papers after my retirement but inevitably most were review articles or retrospective surveys. As alluded to earlier, the most important of these was a survey conducted with colleagues here and in South Africa of data gathered between 1990 and 2014. Statistical analysis showed a strong correlation between the total mortality of 133 FH homozygotes during the 25 years of follow-up and their level of cholesterol on treatment, the latter reflecting the combined effects of lipoprotein apheresis and lipid-lowering drugs such as statins and ezetimibe (Figure 1).[2] Patients with an on-treatment serum cholesterol greater than 15·1 mmol/L, had a hazard ratio for total mortality of 11.5 compared with those with an on-treatment cholesterol of less than 8·1 mmol/L. When compared with the latter those with on-treatment cholesterol of 8·1–15·1 mmol/L had a hazard ratio of 3·6. These differences were statistically significant and remained so after adjustments for confounding factors. Significant differences between the three categories of on-treatment serum total cholesterol (90% of which was LDL cholesterol) were also evident for cardiovascular deaths and major adverse cardiovascular events. Hence, reducing the very high levels of serum cholesterol of FH homozygotes, even to levels that are far from ideal, had a markedly beneficial effect on their long term prognosis. In the future, more stringent reductions in cholesterol should provide even greater benefits.

This paper was published more than 40 years after we first described of the use of plasma exchange to treat homozygous FH. The fact that it took so long to confirm the life-prolonging efficacy of this novel approach underlines the rarity and refractory nature of the disorder and illustrates the difficulties of obtaining statistically significant proof when

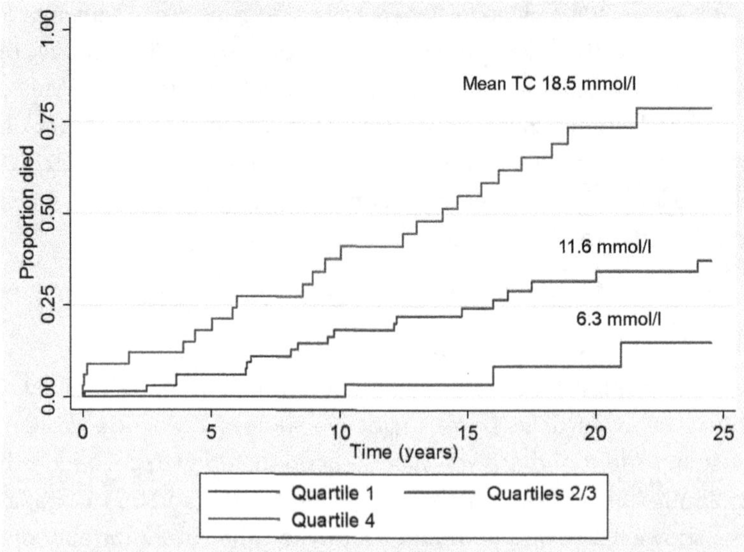

Figure 1. Survival in homozygous familial hypercholesterolaemia according to the on-treatment level of serum cholesterol, showing the proportion of patients who died during 25 years of follow-up. The average total cholesterol (TC) levels in quartiles 1, 2+3, and 4 are shown.

Source: Reproduced from Ref. 2, by permission of Oxford University Press.

a randomised controlled clinical trial is deemed unethical, as was the case here.

The Nobel Prize

I have long had an academic interest in how Nobel Prize winners are chosen and, in 2012, I edited a book *Nobel Prizes that Changed Medicine* that depicted my top 15 of the 100 Nobel Prizes in Physiology or Medicine awarded between 1901 and 2009.[3] The sequel, *Pioneers of Medicine Without a Nobel Prize*,[4] was published 2 years later and described what I considered was an equally remarkable group of individuals who have not received it. As discussed by Norrby[5] the selection process for the Prize in Physiology or Medicine is extremely rigorous but it is not perfect. For example, Oswald Avery's discovery in 1944 of DNA as the carrier of heredity was a major achievement yet despite being nominated 46 times he died without being awarded the Nobel Prize. The latter is never awarded posthumously.

As I have argued elsewhere[6] there are simply not enough Nobel Prizes to reward all those who have made major discoveries in biomedical science. The Prize in Physiology or Medicine is limited to three laureates annually, which means that hard and difficult choices have to be made every year by the Nobel Assembly of the Karolinska Institute in Stockholm. Recently, there has been a distinct bias towards rewarding basic scientific discoveries in preference to clinically related ones.

Prominent Non-Recipients of the Nobel Prize

Many believe that Boyer and Cohen's development of the cloning of recombinant DNA in the 1970s[4] deserves a Nobel Prize. This discovery resulted in an explosion of knowledge and an understanding of human genetics that has benefitted all aspects of clinical medicine.

It is ironic that the spread of the hepatitis C virus was unwittingly facilitated by the use of blood transfusions. The latter procedure has saved countless lives but was also responsible for transmitting disease to millions of people. Working at the National Institutes of Health and the Chiron Corporation, respectively, Harvey Alter and Michael Houghton[4] discovered the hepatitis C virus and developed assays that eliminated the risk of transmitting all forms of viral hepatitis by blood transfusions. These achievements earned them a Lasker Award in 2000 and some argue that they also deserve a Nobel Prize.

Mark Twain stressed the importance of primacy in any discovery and Akira Endo's discovery of the cholesterol-lowering properties of *Penicillium citrinium*[4] was as much a first as was Alexander Fleming's discovery of the antibiotic properties of penicillin. Fleming was awarded the Nobel Prize but Endo, "whose discovery of statins changed the world,"[7] lacks similar recognition despite the fact that the scientific importance of his discovery and its benefit to mankind in reducing morbidity and mortality from atherosclerotic cardiovascular disease clearly fulfil the criteria stipulated in Alfred Nobel's will for the award of the Prize.[8]

Current Trends in Medical Research

A recent development is the use of Mendelian randomisation and genome-wide association studies (GWAS), which provide invaluable information on whether correlations between biomarkers and disease are causal. This raises the question of whether future advances arising from GWAS might be eligible for consideration by the Nobel Assembly. Another development has been the emergence of translational research, which aims to facilitate the conversion of basic science discoveries into clinically relevant advances in investigation and treatment. A classic example, which occurred long before the term was coined, was Fleming's serendipitous but crucial observation of the contaminated culture plate, which would have remained of purely academic interest if Florey and Chain had not subsequently devised a means of producing penicillin in sufficient quantity and purity for clinical use. The current enthusiasm for translational research is not shared by the Nobel laureates Goldstein and Brown who consider that "Individual curiosity driven science has been replaced by large consortia dedicated to the proposition that gathering vast amounts of correlative data will somehow provide the answer to life's fundamental questions."[9]

The challenge facing the Nobel Foundation is how to cope with the changing face of biomedical research, especially when there are scores of authors of a crucial publication. In this situation it may be virtually impossible to decide which three of the individuals involved were responsible for a potential Nobel Prize-winning discovery. It is also questionable whether Nobel's wishes have always been carried out in the spirit he intended — in particular, is too much emphasis placed on the scientific quality of a discovery and not enough on the benefit it confers on mankind? One way of resolving this issue would be to treat the Physiology and Medicine components of the Prize as separate entities. Thus, the Prize in Physiology would be awarded for basic scientific research whereas the Prize in Medicine would be reserved for advances in diagnosis, therapeutics, and the clinical applications of translational research. This would double the number of potential recipients and help redress the perceived bias against clinically-related discoveries. Considering that the first Prize in Physiology or Medicine was awarded in 1901 it is remarkable that the selection process has survived virtually unchanged. But if change does come in Stockholm, one must hope that it will not compromise the Nobel Prize's reputation for recognising excellence.

Doctor of Science

Coming down to earth back in London, I was awarded an Imperial Doctor of Science degree in Metabolic Medicine in 2014 with the citation "for published work of an exceptional standard containing original contributions to the advancement of knowledge and learning which has given the candidate international distinction in his field of study," in other words for publishing rather than perishing. The Postgraduate Graduation Day Ceremonies took place in a packed Albert Hall and mine was one of the last of a large number of degrees presented that afternoon. This meant a very long wait before it was my turn to climb onto the dais wearing a purple and white gown and Tudor velvet hat to receive my DSc from Baroness Manningham-Buller, the Chair of the Court and Council of Imperial College (and ex-director of MI5). Afterwards I celebrated with my long-suffering supporters in the audience, namely my wife and our two daughters.

References

1. Lewis Sir Thomas. The Harveian Oration on "Clinical Science." *Br Med J* 1933;**ii**:717–22.
2. Thompson GR, Blom DJ, Marais AD *et al.* Survival in homozygous familial hypercholesterolaemia is determined by the on-treatment level of serum cholesterol. *Eur Heart J* 2018;**39**:1162–8.
3. Thompson G (ed.). *Nobel Prizes that changed Medicine*. London: Imperial College Press, 2012.
4. Thompson G (ed.). *Pioneers of Medicine without a Nobel Prize*. London: Imperial College Press, 2014.
5. Norrby E. *Nobel Prizes and Life Sciences.* Singapore: World Scientific Publishing Co, 2010.
6. Thompson GR. The Nobel dilemma: To reward scientific discovery or benefit to mankind? *QJM.* 2016;**109**:513–4.
7. Brown MS, Goldstein JL. A tribute to Akira Endo, discoverer of a "Penicillin" for cholesterol. *Atheroscler. Suppl.* 2004;**5**:13–16.

8. "Full text of Alfred Nobel's will." *Nobelprize.org*. Nobel media AB 2013. Web. 19 February 2015. http://www.nobelprize.org/alfred_nobel/will/will-full.html.
9. Goldstein JL, Brown MS. A golden era of Nobel laureates, *Science* 2012; **338**:1033–4.

19 The Expanding Scene of Lipid-Lowering Agents

Statins and the Post-Statin Era

This penultimate chapter reappraises the current role of statins in relation to the prevention and treatment of atherosclerotic cardiovascular disease, and it also describes the remarkable advances in lipid-lowering drug therapy that have occurred during the past decade.

The only drugs available to treat hyperlipidaemia in the 1960s were clofibrate and cholestyramine and the subsequent development of modern lipid-lowering compounds transformed our ability to treat patients effectively. The therapeutic revolution that took place is analogous to the one that followed the introduction of antibiotics, and was initiated in the 1970s by the discovery of the LDL receptor and promulgated by the discovery of compactin and its successors. Statins remain the first-line treatment for most patients with or at high risk for cardiovascular disease but the post-statin era of lipid-lowering drugs currently under development holds great promise for the management of severe lipid disorders that are refractory to statins, especially homozygous FH.

Statins and ezetimibe

A survey of more than 1,000 UK patients with the less severe, heterozygous form of FH in 1999 showed that their mortality from coronary heart disease had halved since 1992, reflecting the widespread use of statins to treat this particular group of patients from 1989 onwards, when simvastatin was first licensed in Britain.[1] One possible explanation for the magnitude of this decrease over such a short space of time is that FH heterozygotes, whose main risk factor is a raised LDL, respond better to lipid-lowering therapy than do non-FH patients with a lower LDL cholesterol but with various other risk factors.[2]

If one considers the situation in the population at large, only 1:250 of whom have FH, it has been estimated that the major modifiable risk factors, namely raised serum cholesterol, smoking, and high blood pressure, account for 45%, 29% and 22%, respectively, of all myocardial infarcts (heart attacks).[3] Hence, it is important to examine temporal changes in all three risk factors when trying to explain changes in cardiovascular mortality. In an analysis of the large decrease in coronary mortality in England and Wales that occurred between 1981 and 2000, public health workers in Liverpool calculated the number of deaths prevented or postponed by specific cardiac interventions and risk factor changes for each of those years.[4] The results suggest that approximately 42% of the decrease was due to cardiological procedures, both medical and surgical, and the remainder to reductions in risk factors. Of the latter, 48% was due to decreased smoking and only 10% each to decreases in cholesterol and blood pressure. Subsequently, a similar study was conducted in the USA to investigate the decrease in coronary mortality that had occurred over there during the same period.[5] As in Britain, just under 50% of the reduction in mortality was attributable to medical or surgical interventions, and the remainder reflected risk factor changes. However, in contrast to Britain, decreased smoking accounted for only 12% of the reduction in coronary mortality, whereas decreases in serum cholesterol and blood pressure contributed to 24% and 20% of the reduction, respectively. The finding that decreases in serum cholesterol made a larger contribution to the reduction in coronary heart disease mortality in the USA than in Britain presumably reflected the earlier introduction and greater use of statins over there at that time.

Interestingly, the latest British Heart Foundation statistics[6] show that prescriptions for lipid-lowering drugs in England, predominantly statins, increased from 1,066,000 in 1991 to 70,957,000 in 2016, a staggering 70-fold increment! The number of coronary artery bypass graft (CABG) operations remained stable but percutaneous coronary interventions (PCI) increased 10-fold. Over this 25 years period the UK death rate from coronary heart disease in men and women of all ages decreased by 63%, the presumption being that the increased use of statins and revascularisation procedures (CABG and PCI) both contributed to this outcome. However, the rate of decrease in mortality and morbidity from cardiovascular disease has slowed markedly since 2015, possibly reflecting recent increases in the prevalence of obesity and diabetes in the population.

Statins have proved to be highly effective in young and middle-aged subjects at high risk, including those with FH, but whether they should be used across a wider spectrum of ages and risk categories is debatable. Caveats about their cost no longer apply now that all the statins currently licensed in the UK are generic and much cheaper than before. The basic cost to the NHS of 1 year's treatment at the start of 2019 ranged from only £8–32 for atorvastatin 10 mg daily to £33 for rosuvastatin 40 mg daily. The majority of patients with hyperlipidaemia, including many of those with FH, respond adequately to statin therapy alone or combined with the cholesterol absorption blocker ezetimibe. Addition of the latter results in an additional 15% reduction in LDL cholesterol and enables a lower dose of statin to be used if desired. However, there is a minority of subjects whose LDL cholesterol remains high despite treatment or who are apparently intolerant of these drugs.

Statin intolerance

The question of statin intolerance has been a recurring topic of sometimes misleading comment in the lay press over the last few years. In a recent authoritative and detailed analysis of all the published evidence from clinical trials Collins *et al.* estimated that statins cause symptomatic intolerance, notably muscle pain, in about 50–100 patients per 10,000 treated for 5 years (0.5–1%).[7] However, placebo-controlled randomised trials have shown that almost all of the adverse symptoms attributed to statin therapy in clinical practice are not actually caused by it (i.e. they represent misattribution). A possible explanation for this is the nocebo effect, the inverse of the placebo effect, a phenomenon that refers to adverse events that reflect subjective expectations of harm from a drug. The latter can be driven by many factors including warnings about adverse effects by clinicians when prescribing a drug, and misinformation in the media about its dangers. According to Tobert and Newman the nocebo effect is the most likely explanation for the high rate of muscle and other symptoms attributed to statins in observational studies and clinical practice, because in randomized controlled trials the frequency of these symptoms was similar in the statin and placebo groups.[8] Self-diagnosed statin-intolerant patients usually tolerate statins under double-blind conditions, which suggests that genuine statin intolerance is much less common than is claimed. But it does exist and when it occurs is sometimes due to loss of function mutations of genes enabling the transport of statins from the blood into the liver. This results in high blood levels of statins, which predispose to side-effects such as myopathy.

Recently, it has become apparent that statins may induce diabetes in some individuals, especially if they already have impaired glucose tolerance. The mechanism of this effect is uncertain but seems to be related to the potency and dose of the statin concerned, perhaps reflecting the extent to which the latter decreases cholesterol synthesis in insulin-secreting pancreatic islet cells. Hence, in subjects with or at risk of developing diabetes it is prudent to use as low a dose as possible of a low intensity statin, supplemented if necessary with ezetimibe, which is not diabetogenic.

PCSK9 inhibitors

For genuinely statin-intolerant individuals and for patients with FH, a new class of lipid-lowering agent has recently become available. These are the PCSK9 inhibitors, monoclonal antibodies that reduce the rate of degradation of LDL receptors by PCSK9 and thereby promote receptor-mediated LDL uptake by the liver; these are given by injection every 2–4 weeks at a cost of approximately £4,500 annually. Their LDL-lowering effect is equivalent to that of a high dose, potent statin and is additive to the effect of the latter.

The discovery of PCSK9 inhibitors is a fascinating one and, like the discovery of the LDL receptor, resulted from studies of patients with rare genetic mutations. Proprotein convertase subtilisin kexin 9, to give PCSK9 its full name, is the ninth member of a family of human proteolytic enzymes, one of its functions being to induce the lysosomal degradation (biological destruction) of the LDL receptor. In 2003, hypercholesterolaemia due to an increase in LDL levels was reported in members of 2 French families with a gain of function mutation of PCSK9.[9] Two years later it was reported that loss of function mutations of the gene were associated with subnormal levels of LDL and a markedly reduced risk of coronary heart disease.[9] This pointed to the potential of PCSK9 inhibition as a means of treating hypercholesterolaemia, either as a substitute for statins in statin-intolerant subjects or as an adjunct in statin-refractory subjects, given that the ability of statins to upregulate the LDL receptor and thereby lower LDL is limited by the increase in PCSK9 levels that they induce.[10]

Current pharmacological approaches to inhibiting PCSK9 are humanised monoclonal antibodies (mAbs), two of which, evolocumab and alirocumab, are licensed for use in patients with or at high risk of developing atherosclerotic CVD. A recent meta-analysis of 24 randomised trials in over 10,000 subjects given various doses of evolocumab or alirocumab by subcutaneous injection once or twice monthly showed a mean reduction in LDL cholesterol of 47%.[11] Data from individual trials of evolocumab showed reductions in LDL cholesterol of 60% at maximum dosage; mAb-related decreases were similar irrespective of whether patients did or did not have heterozygous FH[12,13] or of whether or not they were receiving concomitant statin therapy.[14] Two open label trials of evolocumab showed that doses of 140 mg every 2 weeks or 420 mg monthly for 11 months reduced LDL cholesterol by 61% from 3.1 to 1.2 mmol/L and halved the risk of CV events.[15]

In the meta-analysis referred to above levels of Lp(a) were reduced by 25%, which is roughly half the reduction achieved in LDL cholesterol. This illustrates one of the limitations of PCSK9 mAbs and probably reflects the fact that Lp(a) is not catabolised by the LDL receptor pathway. Another limitation is their relatively low efficacy in patients with homozygous FH, reductions in LDL cholesterol on evolocumab averaging only 23%.[16]

From the practical point of view PCSK9 mAbs clearly have enormous potential as an adjunct to statins and ezetimibe in the treatment of patients with heterozygous FH and as an alternative in statin-refractory or intolerant patients with CVD. However, their usefulness in homozygous FH is much less and often they will complement rather than replace lipoprotein apheresis.

The most recent development in the field of PCSK9 inhibition is Inclisiran, a small interfering RNA (siRNA) nucleotide molecule that prevents the translation of PCSK9 in the liver.[17] Given twice yearly it achieves a 50% reduction in LDL cholesterol over and above the effect of background statin/ezetimibe therapy. Currently this compound is undergoing long-term phase three trials which, if successful, might eventually lead to it supplanting the anti-PCSK9 monoclonal antibodies in current use. The availability of the twin LDL receptor-upregulating options of statins and PCSK9 inhibitors means that, finances permitting, raised LDL cholesterol levels can be lowered very effectively in the majority of eligible patients exhibiting some degree of residual LDL receptor activity.

Lomitapide

Lomitapide, a microsomal triglyceride transfer protein (MTP) inhibitor, is used to treat extreme forms of hypercholesterolaemia such as homozygous FH,[18] and hypertriglyceridaemia, specifically familial hyperchylomicronaemia. Unlike all the other lipid-lowering drugs described above lomitapide inhibits the secretion of apoB-containing lipoproteins and does not depend upon LDL receptor activity. In essence it induces an iatrogenic form of αβ-lipoproteinaemia (recessively inherited MTP deficiency) and has the latter's drawback of causing a fatty liver. It remains to be seen whether this will eventually lead to hepatic fibrosis but in patients with those extreme forms of hyperlipidaemia, which predispose to premature atherosclerosis and acute pancreatitis, respectively, this seems a risk worth taking.

Evinacumab

The latest kid on the block is Evinacumab, a monoclonal antibody to angiopoietin-like 3 (ANGPTL3) that has been shown in a preliminary study to decrease LDL cholesterol by 49% in FH homozygotes.[19] Other studies show that the mechanism is independent of the LDL receptor pathway and involves increased activity of lipoprotein lipase. Evinacumab does not induce a fatty liver but further studies are needed before its therapeutic potential and safety can be fully evaluated.

The Cholesterol Controversy and the Anti-Statin Lobby

Nearly 40 years ago Nick Myant, a scrupulously honest scientist, commented on the need for objectivity when considering the role of cholesterol in ischaemic heart disease.[20] "It should not be necessary to refer here to the need for balance and objectivity in the sifting of evidence, something that has been taken for granted by the scientific community for about 300 years. Nevertheless, it is a fact that the very word 'cholesterol' tends to arouse emotional reactions that cloud judgement ... The reason for this state of affairs is, of course, the link thought to exist between cholesterol and a disease so serious and widespread that it is difficult not to feel strongly about it ... I see no advantage in adopting an evangelistic approach, since the question will ultimately be settled by the methods of science. It seems to me that those engaged in the current controversy should try to emulate Darwin, one of whose endearing traits was a horror of being unfair to his opponents ... he kept a special notebook for facts that went against his theory — because he found that he tended to forget them!"

The controversy over cholesterol may have died down but is certainly not extinct. As Francis Bacon pointed out over 400 years ago, "If a man will begin with certainties, he shall end in doubts; but if he will be content to begin with doubts, he shall end in certainties."[21] However, there will always be some who begin with doubts and never relinquish them, epitomized by the International Network of Cholesterol Skeptics. One of their mottos is "The growth of knowledge depends entirely on disagreement," which they put into practice by publishing letters and review articles with pejorative titles such as "LDL-C does not cause cardiovascular disease."[22] In these they criticise others for falsifying the lipid hypothesis by using misleading statistics and ignoring contradictory findings but they never provide any experimental data supporting an alternative explanation for the aetiology of atherosclerosis. Perhaps another of their mottos should be "If you throw enough mud at the wall, some of it will stick."

Nowadays the anti-cholesterol movement increasingly manifests itself in anti-statin lobbying, with potentially harmful consequences for those whose continuing health depends upon taking these compounds. A recent article in the *European Heart Journal* drew attention to and roundly criticised a recent Franco-German television programme called "The Big Bluff," which stated that there was no relationship between blood cholesterol levels and cardiovascular disease. Consequently, the programme advised viewers to avoid having their cholesterol levels checked and to discontinue taking statins.[23] In their rebuttal, the authors of the *European Heart Journal* article emphasised the strength of the evidence causally linking raised LDL cholesterol and cardiovascular disease and the beneficial effects of statins on both. They also cited a recent Danish study, which demonstrated that negative statin-related news stories from newspapers and magazines, radio and TV stations, and internet websites were associated with an increase in the proportion of patients discontinuing statin therapy and with significant increases in the risks of myocardial infarction and cardiovascular death compared with those who continued to take statins.[24]

References

1. Scientific Steering Committee on behalf of the Simon Broome Register Group. Mortality in treated heterozygous familial hypercholesterolaemia: Implications for clinical management. *Atherosclerosis* 1999;**142**:105–12.
2. Thompson GR. Atherosclerosis in cholesterol-fed rabbits and in homozygous and heterozygous LDL receptor-deficient humans. *Atherosclerosis* 2018;**276**:148–54.
3. Yusuf S, Hawken S, Ounpuu S *et al*. Effect of potentially modifiable risk factors associated with myocardial infarction in 52 countries (the INTERHEART study): Case-control study. *Lancet* 2004;**364**:937–52.
4. Unal B, Critchley JA, Capewell S. Explaining the decline in coronary heart disease mortality in England and Wales between 1981 and 2000. *Circulation* 2004;**109**:1101–7.
5. Ford ES, Ajani UA, Croft JB *et al*. Explaining the decline in U.S. deaths from coronary disease, 1980–2000. *N Engl J Med* 2007;**356**:2388–98.
6. British Heart Foundation Heart and Circulatory Diseases Statistics 2018. www.bhf.org.uk.
7. Collins R, Reith C, Emberson J *et al*. Interpretation of the evidence for the efficacy and safety of statin therapy. Lancet 2016;**388**:2532–61.
8. Tobert JA, Newman CB. The nocebo effect in the context of statin intolerance. J Clin Lipidol 2016;**10**:739–47.
9. Lambert G. Unravelling the functional significance of PCSK9. *Curr Opin Lipidol* 2007;**18**:304–9.
10. Seidah NG, Prat A. The biology and therapeutic targeting of the proprotein convertases. *Nat Rev Drug Discov* 2012;**11**:367–83.
11. Navarese EP, Kolodzieiczak M, Schulze V *et al*. Effects of proprotein convertase subtilisin/kexin type 9 antibodies in adults with hypercholesterolemia: A systematic review and meta-analysis. *Ann Intern Med* 2015;**163**:40–51.

12. Raal FJ, Stein EA, Dufour R *et al.* PCSK9 inhibition with evolocumab (AMG 145) in heterozygous familial hypercholesterolaemia (RUTHERFORD-2): a randomised, double-blind, placebo-controlled trial. *Lancet* 2015;**385**:331–40.
13. Koren MJ, Scott R, Kim JB *et al.* Efficacy, safety, and tolerability of a monoclonal antibody to proprotein convertase subtilisin/kexin type 9 as monotherapy in patients with hypercholesterolaemia (MENDEL): A randomised, double-blind, placebo-controlled, phase 2 study. *Lancet* 2012;**380**:1995–2006.
14. Blom D, Hala T, Bolognese M *et al.* A 52-week placebo-controlled trial of evolocumab in hyperlipidemia. *N Engl J Med* 2014;**370**:1809–19.
15. Sabatine MS, Giugliano RP, Wiviott SD *et al.* Efficacy and safety of evolocumab in reducing lipids and cardiovascular events. *N Engl J Med* 2015; **372**:1500–9.
16. Raal FJ, Hovingh GK, Blom DJ *et al.* Long-term treatment with evolocumab added to conventional drug therapy, with or without apheresis, in 106 homozygous familial hypercholesterolaemia patients: An interim subset analysis of the open-label TAUSSIG study. *Lancet Diabetes Endocrinol* 2017;**5**:280–90.
17. Ray KK, Stoekenbroek RM, Kallend D *et al.* Effect of an siRNA therapeutic targeting PCSK9 on atherogenic lipoproteins. *Circulation* 2018;**138**:1304–16.
18. Cuchel M, Meagher EA, du Toit Theron H *et al.* Efficacy and safety of a microsomal triglyceride transfer protein inhibitor in patients with homozygous familial hypercholesterolaemia: A single-arm, open-label, phase 3 study. *Lancet* 2013;**381**:40–6.
19. Gaudet G, Gipe DA, Pordy R *et al.* ANGPTL3 inhibition in homozygous familial hypercholesterolemia. *N Eng J Med* 2017;**377**:296–7.
20. Myant NB. *The Biology of Cholesterol and Related Steroids.* London: Heinemann, 1981.
21. Francis B. *The Advancement of Learning*, First published in 1605; revised edition. New York: Modern Library, 2001.
22. Ravnskov U, de Lorgeril M, Diamond DM *et al.* LDL-C does not cause cardiovascular disease: A comprehensive review of the current literature. *Expert Rev Clin Pharmacol* 2018;**11**:959–70.
23. Schiele F, Kristensen SD. The anti-statin lobby strikes again: Time to set the record straight. *Eur Heart J* 2018;**39**:335–6.
24. Nielsen SF, Nordestgaard BG. Negative statin-related news stories decrease statin persistence and increase myocardial infarction and cardiovascular mortality: A nationwide prospective cohort study. *Eur Heart J* 2016;**37**:908–16.

20 Epilogue

The Lipid Hypothesis: Q.E.D

Anitschkow put the diametrically opposite point of view to that of the cholesterol sceptics more than a century ago in St. Petersburg when he stated "Without cholesterol there can be no atherosclerosis." The evidence summarised in this book strongly supports this premise and vindicates my decision "to take the road less travelled by" in my research career. Accepting that the lipid hypothesis-basis of atherosclerosis has been proved, it follows that lowering cholesterol by diet, drugs, or apheresis is a *sine qua non* if atherosclerotic cardiovascular disease is to be prevented in subjects with a raised LDL cholesterol, especially those with FH. A Dutch study has shown that statin treatment of heterozygotes reduces their risk of myocardial infarction to that of the general population whereas if left untreated their risk of premature death from cardiovascular disease remains much higher.[1] Advances in genetic diagnosis have led to concerted campaigns by HEART UK, the International Atherosclerosis Society, and other organisations to identify affected individuals by screening and offer them appropriate treatment. As yet the latter does not include gene therapy but that must be the ultimate goal, at least for homozygotes.

Doctors and Flyfishing

Allusions to flyfishing in the medical literature are scarce and are often light-hearted. For example in the Christmas 1998 edition of the *BMJ*, a group of physicians and surgeons compared the ability of five dry flies to catch brown trout on a chalk stream in the Collaborative Randomised and

Controlled Kennet Piscatorial Options Trial (CRACKPOT).[2] The study was approved by the public bar Ethics Committee of the Riverside Inn, Canonbie, Dumfriesshire. The investigators found that a Cinnamon Sedge was the most successful fly and a Black Gnat the least successful and concluded that prolongation of doctors' leisure time due to the use of unproductive trout flies had resource implications for the NHS!

Perhaps the best known medically qualified author who fished was Richard Gordon (the late Dr. Richard Ostlere), who wrote *Doctor in the House*. He described his piscatorial exploits in his autobiographical *Fifty Years a Fisherman*,[3] and although much of the book is devoted to his experiences as a ship's doctor and an anaesthetist and to his impressions of the actors and actresses who starred in the various *Doctor* films, one glimpses his sense of priorities when he writes "having a rod on the River Kennet I sought a job at Oxford University" and "without interrupting the trout season I married my assistant."

Taking a leaf out of his book, I will recount a memorable experience I had on the River Test in Hampshire a few years ago. It was a humid and overcast afternoon in late September and the fishing season was nearly over. I had caught nothing all day and was slowly walking up the river towards the top of the beat when I saw a tiny disturbance in the water close to the brick wall that shored up the far bank. I knew from experience that large trout tended to lie there waiting for flies to be carried downstream by the current but I also knew that they were nigh impossible to catch.

It was difficult to reach the opposite bank from where I was standing because my back cast was constrained by a regiment of head-high reeds behind me. I therefore set about beating them down with a stick until I had just enough room to cast a fly to the far bank. After several attempts I managed to put my fly, a small Red Sedge, over the spot where I'd earlier seen that dimple. Suddenly up from the depths came a dark shape like a submarine surfacing, the fly disappeared, I struck, the line tightened, and my rod bent ominously. I played the fish carefully for 5–10 minutes, worried by its size and the abundant weed. However, all went well and I netted and landed it successfully. It was a beautifully proportioned brown trout with a magnificent tail and pristine fins, and looked to all intents and purposes to be a wild fish, not a stocked one. It weighed 7 lb and although it was no record breaker it was the largest brown trout caught that year on the stretch of the Test that I fish and the biggest one I had ever caught.

Stuffed, the fish now resides in a bow-fronted case with its provenance inscribed in traditional 18 carat gold lettering on the glass. It evokes for me Isaac Walton's description of angling as "a rest to his mind, a cheerer of his spirits, a diverter of sadness, a calmer of unquiet thoughts, a moderator of passions, a procurer of contentedness." The late Hugh Falkus, another famous but contemporary fisherman, expressed similar sentiments more succinctly and in modern parlance in the title of his book, *Some of It Was Fun*.[4] In it he describes waiting to see if a trout would rise in a stream he could see from the courtyard of the French chateau where he was about to be shot as a spy. His Spitfire had crashed nearby but he had taken off from RAF Duxford in such a hurry on that morning in June 1940 that he was still in his pyjamas, raising dire suspicions about his identity in the humourless minds of his Nazi captors. Happily he was saved from that fate by a senior officer and gentleman of the Wehrmacht and became a prisoner for the remainder of the war.

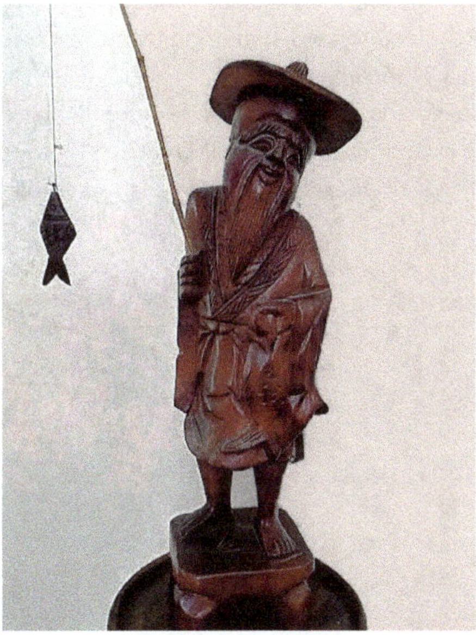

Figure 1. Wooden statue of a Chinese fisherman (gift from Nikolai Naoumov and Rossi Naoumova).

Conclusion

All things must come to an end and "Some of it was fun" is an apt description of my medical career; highlights were investigating the relationship between haemoglobin C and malaria in Ghana, vitamin D absorption in London and Boston, apoB metabolism in Houston and Montreal, and establishing the roles of apheresis and statins in the management of FH at the Hammersmith. The same description also applies to the R and R time I spent fishing in various parts of the world. To paraphrase the Chinese proverb embodied by Figure 1, "Give a man a fish and make him happy for a day, teach him how to fish and make him happy for the rest of his days." Speaking of happiness perhaps the greatest source of this for me has been the many friends, colleagues, and patients I acquired during my medical and piscatorial pursuits. Sadly, some of them are now dead but not forgotten and their memory lives on in this book.

References

1. Versmissen J, Oosterveer DM, Yazdanpanath M *et al.* Efficacy of statins in familial hypercholesterolaemia: a long term cohort study. *BMJ* 2008; **337**:a2423. doi: 10.1136/bmj.a2423.
2. Britton BJ, Grimley Evans J, Potter JM. Does the fly matter? The CRACKPOT study in evidence based trout fishing. *BMJ* 1998;**317**:1678–80.
3. Gordon R. *Fifty Years a Fisherman*. London: Harrap, 1985.
4. Falkus H. *Some of It Was Fun*. Ellesmere: Medlar Press, 2003.

Index

A
Accra, 14, 17–19, 24–25
Alamo, 40, 43
albumin, 50, 118
alirocumab, 181
Alter, Harvey, 173
Amarillo, 42
American War of Independence, 152
angiopoietin-like 3 (ANGPTL3), 182
Anitschkow, Nikolai N., 70, 187
anti-cholesterol movement, 183
aortic root, 124
aortic stenosis, 125
apheresis, 117, 121–122, 124–125, 190
apo(a), 125
apoB, 40, 85, 190
Apstein, Carl, S., 122
Ardvreck Castle, 135
army, 9, 22
Astrup, Paul, 69
atheromatous plaque, 123–124
atherosclerosis, 33, 37, 46, 50, 75, 77, 187
Atherosclerosis Discussion Group (ADG), 79–80, 82
atorvastatin, 90, 179
Avery, Oswald, 172

B
Bacon, Francis, 183
Bahamas, 149–151
Ball, Keith, 49
Band, George, 7
Bayer, 90
BBC TV debate, 48
Berg, Kare, 125
Big Bend National Park, 42
Blankenhorn, David, 107
bonefish, 151, 154, 156–157
bonefish flats, 154
Booth, Chris, 24, 27, 30–31, 33, 38, 45, 73, 113
Bordier, Philippe, 31
Boston, 31, 33–34, 37–38, 58, 62, 86, 190
Boston marathon, 143, 146
Boyd, George, 56–57
Boyer, Herbert, 173
British Army, 1

British Association of Lipid Disorders (BALD), 109
British Atherosclerosis Discussion Group, 107
British Atherosclerosis Society (BAS), 79–80
British Cardiac Society, 56–57, 67–68, 97
British Cardiovascular Society, 57
British Heart Foundation, 141, 144, 178
British Hyperlipidaemia Association (BHA), 97, 109–110
British Loyalists, 151
Brompton Hospital, 52
Bronte-Stewart, Brian, 57
Brown, Greg, 106–107
Brown, Michael, 32, 53, 61–62, 111, 126, 141
brown trout, 187–188
Bruce, Sandison, 133–134, 138
Buchwald, Henry, 72
Bywaters, Eric, 12

C

Cambridge, 80, 82, 107
Campbell, Moran, 27
camping, 34, 41
Canada, 130
cardiac arrest, 142, 146–147
cardiopulmonary resuscitation, 146
cardiovascular disease, 38
Carlson, Lars, 68
Casualty, 6, 13, 23
Censors' Room, 13
cerivastatin, 90
cholesterol, 33, 46, 52, 56, 77, 122, 149, 183, 187
cholesterol controversy, 55
cholesterol-lowering medication, 100, 102
Cholesterol Treatment Trialists' Collaboration (CTTC), 113
cholestyramine, 71–72, 105, 177
climbing, 7
clofibrate, 69, 108, 177
Cohen, Stanley, 173
Cold War, 159, 164, 168
colestipol, 105
Collins, Rory, 112
Committee on Medical Aspects (COMA), 47, 49, 75, 77
compactin, 87, 177
Cornforth, John, 59
coronary angiography, 71
coronary artery bypass, 51–52
coronary artery bypass graft (CABG), 178
coronary artery disease, 145
coronary heart disease, 33, 46, 49, 56, 77, 146
creatine kinase MB, 142–143
Crone, Christian, 69
Crozier Street, 5–6
cutaneous xanthomas, 70
Cuthbertson, Cuth, 79

D

Dallas, 27, 38, 62, 88, 120
Darwin, 183
Davey Smith, George, 100–101
Davies, Michael, 106–107
de Gennes, Jean-Luc, 117
dextran sulphate adsorption, 119
dietary lipids, 77
DNA, 172–173
Doctor of Science, 175

double filtration plasmapheresis (DFPP), 118
Dowling, Hermon, 33, 37, 68, 134
Downing College, 107
Downside, 2–3
duck shooting, 39

E

East Litza, 162, 166
Eisenberg, Shlomo, 68
Endo, Akira, 87–88, 90, 93, 173
England, 38
epidemiology, 58
Eskimos, 81
European Atherosclerosis Society, 97, 107, 125
European Society for Clinical Investigation (ESCI), 68
Evans, Willie, 11
evinacumab, 182
evolocumab, 181
Exuma, 149, 151
ezetimibe, 110, 122, 171, 179–180

F

falciparum malaria, 21–22
Falkus, Hugh, 189
familial hypercholesterolaemia (FH), 50, 52, 60, 187, 190
familial hyperchylomicronaemia, 182
FH homozygotes, 50, 171
final viva, 12–13
Firehole River, 34
fish, 3, 190
fisherman, 1
Fisher's Pond, 2
fish farm, 133, 163
fishing, 1–2
Fleming, Alexander, 93, 173
Florey, Sir Howard, 79
fluvastatin, 90
Flyfishers' Club, 139
flyfishing, 2, 155, 187
Food and Drug Administration (FDA), 89
fractional catabolic rates (FCR), 121–122
Fraser, Russell, 12
Frazer, Alistair, 59, 61
Frazer, Francis, 65
Fredrickson, Don, 33, 38, 48, 63
Fredrickson, Donald, 61
Freetown, Sierra Leone, 17
French, John, 79
Frost, Robert, 54, 60

G

Gaines, Charles, 161–162
Gairdner International Award, 93
Galveston, 40
gastroenterology, 31, 37, 45
George Town, 150–151, 153
German Lipoprotein Apheresis Registry, 126
Ghana, 14, 17, 21–25, 27, 30, 190
Ghana Army, 14, 18
Glaxo, 79
Goldstein, Joe, 32, 53, 62, 110–111, 141
Goodman, 122
Goodpasture's syndrome, 118
Goodwin, John, 68
Gorbachev, Mikhail, 159
Gordon, Richard, 188
Gotto, Tony, 38–39, 41, 45, 53
Grand Rounds, 32

Gresham, Austin, 80
Grimble, Augustus, 136, 138
Grundy, Scott, 53
guinea worm, 20
Guseran, 130, 133
Guy's Hospital, 12

H

haemoglobin A, 21–23
haemoglobin C, 21–25, 190
haemoglobin S, 21, 23–25
Hammarskjold, Dag, 19
Hammersmith Hospital, 11, 14, 25, 27, 32, 37, 45, 53, 55, 65, 106, 170–171, 190
Hampton, John, 79
Handbook of Hyperlipidaemia, 141
Harvard Medical School, 32
Harveian Oration, 66, 73, 169
Haskins, Tim, 161
Hay, Peter, 136, 138
Heart Protection Study (HPS), 112–113
HEART UK, 109–110, 187
helicopter, 162, 166
HELP, 118
heterozygous FH, 85, 88, 181
high density lipoprotein (HDL), 56, 117
Hi-Ho, 150, 153
Himsworth, Sir Harlold, 58
HMG-CoA reductase, 87
Holland, 11, 106
homozygous FH, 50–51, 70, 88, 117, 121, 171, 181–182
Hôpital Lariboisiere, 31
Horse Guards, 14–15
Houghton, Michael, 173
house officer, 9
Houston, 38, 41–43, 190
Howard, Alan, 107
Hugh Sinclair Memorial Lecture, 81
Hunter, Donald, 11
Hurricane Andrew, 157
hypercholesterolaemia, 87
hyperlipidaemia, 52, 177
hypertrophic cardiomyopathy, 145–146

I

immunoapheresis, 118
Imperial College London, 169
International Atherosclerosis Society, 187
International Network of Cholesterol Skeptics, 183
Inverie, 130, 133
Inverie harbour, 130
Isselbacher, Kurt, 31–32

J

Jagannathan, S. N., 123
Jesus College, 80
John French Memorial Lecture, 80

K

Kaneka, 119
Karolinska Institute, 173
Katz, Saul S., 123
Kennedy, John F., 27
Kennet, 188
Keys, Ancel, 57, 61
Kharlovka, 162, 164–165
Kirkaig, 134, 136–138
Kitchener, 3
Knoydart, 129, 132–133
Knoydart Foundation, 130
Kola Peninsula, 161, 163

Kremlin, 159
Khrushchev, Nikita, 27

L

Labadi Beach, 18
Lagos, Nigeria, 24
Lambeth Hospital, 13
Lasker Award, 93, 173
Latimer, Adrian, 166
Law, Malcolm, 100–101
LDL cholesterol, 181
LDL receptor, 62, 120, 177, 181
LDL turnover, 119
Lehman, Hermann, 26
Leiden University, 22
Leningrad, 160
Levy, Bob, 38, 53, 62, 71
Lewis, Barry, 50, 60
Lewis, Sir Thomas, 60, 169
lipid clinic, 60, 91, 170
lipid hypothesis, 60, 66, 69, 72, 183
lipid-lowering drug, 105, 177–178
lipidology, 33, 58
Lipid Research Clinics (LRC), 38
lipids, 37, 45, 50
lipoprotein, 33, 38, 45
lipoprotein apheresis, 51, 91, 117–118, 126, 171, 181
lipoprotein lipase, 182
Lochinver, 134, 136
lomitapide, 126, 182
London, 4, 14, 24, 27, 37, 52, 65, 152, 190
London marathon, 141, 145
lovastatin, 89–90, 100, 105
low density lipoprotein (LDL), 40, 56, 85, 117
Lp(a), 125–126, 181
LRC Coronary Primary Prevention trial, 78
LRC Primary Prevention Trial, 71
Lucien Award, 85

M

MAAS trial, 106
MacMillan, Harold, 19
Magdalen College, 57, 80
malaria, 20, 22, 24–25, 190
Mallaig, 129, 133
Manningham-Buller, Baroness, 175
Manson, Liz, 142
Massachusetts General Hospital (MGH), 31–33, 38
McIntyre, Neil, 33, 86
McManus, Jim, 33
McMichael, John, 25, 27, 33, 55, 58, 60, 65, 68, 72
MD thesis, 25–26
Medical Research Council (MRC), 31, 47, 51, 58, 60, 170
Medical Research Society (MRS), 30
Mencken, HL, 77–78
Merck, 87, 89, 141
Merryweather, James, 134
Methodist Hospital, 38
mevinolin, 87
Middlesex Hospital, 5, 48
Military Hospital, Accra (*see also* No. 37), 18
Millennium, 161
Milne, Malcolm, 12, 66
Mitchell, Tony, 47, 75, 77
monoclonal antibodies, 180–182
Montreal, 85, 190
Mont Royal, 85
Morris, Jerry, 58
Moscow, 92, 160

MRC Lipid Metabolism Unit, 50, 60
MRCP, 12, 14
Muldoon, 99, 101
Munros, 132
Murmansk, 161, 163
myalgia, 142
Myant Lecture, 109
Myant, Nick, 50–51, 60, 109, 182
myocardial infarction, 47, 75, 145
myopathy, 180
myotoxicity, 90

N

Naoumova, Rossi, 170
National Institutes of Health (NIH), 33, 38, 49, 51, 61–62, 97
National Service, 9
Neale, Graham, 28
Newton, Roger, 90
New York marathon, 144
Nkrumah, Kwame, 19
Nobel Prize, 32, 59, 79, 112, 172–173
nocebo effect, 179–180
North Atlantic Salmon Fund, 134
Northern Territories (NTs), 20

O

Oakley, Celia, 52, 71
Oliver, Michael, 56, 77, 79, 97, 100–101, 106, 108, 113
Oxford, 57, 75, 79

P

Pappworth, Maurice, 58
Paris, 31
Parke-Davis, 90
partial ileal bypass, 72, 105
PCSK9 inhibitors, 180, 182
Peace and Plenty, 152–153
Pekkanen, Juha, 100
penicillin, 6, 79
percutaneous coronary interventions (PCI), 178
Peters, Keith, 72, 118–119
Pickering, George, 57
plasma exchange, 50–51, 70, 86, 117–118, 120, 171
plasmapheresis, 117
Police, 18, 21–22
Popjak, George, 53, 59
Porter, Sir George, 48
Power, Peter, 162–164, 167
pravastatin, 90, 100, 109
progression, 106
pseudo-myocardial infarction, 143

Q

Quebec, 86
Queen Alexandra Military Hospital, 11, 24
Queen's College, 82

R

rabies, 24
rainbow trout, 34
RAMC College, 10, 12
Raphael, Maurice, 71
Red Square, 159
regression, 70, 91, 106
regression trials, 105, 107
Republic of Congo, 20
rhabdomyolysis, 90
Rio Grande, 43
risk factors, 178
Rolle, Will, 152, 155
Rose, Geoffrey, 97
rosuvastatin, 90, 179

Royal Army Medical Corps (RAMC), 3, 10, 12
Royal College of Physicians, 11, 13, 24, 67, 78
Royal Free Hospital, 30, 86
Royal Postgraduate Medical School, 45, 51, 119, 169
Royal Victoria Hospital, 85
rugby, 7
Russia, 159, 161
Rynda, 162, 164

S

salmon, 131, 134, 166
salmon fishing, 162, 164
San Francisco, 34
Sankyo, 88–89
saturated fat, 76–77
saturated fat theory, 46
Scandinavian Simvastatin Survival Study (4S), 107, 141
Scotland, 129
sea trout, 131, 133
Seed, Mary, 125
serotonin, 99
Sgùrr na Cìche, 132
Shaper, Gerry, 68
Shark Channel, 154–155
Sharpey-Schafer, Peter, 8, 55, 65–66
Shepherd, Jim, 109–110
Sherlock, Sheila, 12, 30–31, 66
Shillingford, Jack, 45
sickle cell disease, 21
sickle cell trait, 21–23, 25
Simon Broome Familial Hyperlipidaemia Register, 111
simvastatin, 100, 112, 177
Sinclair, Hugh, 57, 79
Slack, Joan, 80
slaves, 152
small interfering RNA (siRNA), 181
Smith, Elspeth, 80
Smith, Sydney, 67
Sniderman, Allan, 85
Sound of Sleat, 129, 131, 133
Soutar, Anne, 80
South Africa, 57, 171
Soviet Union, 159, 164
splenic infarcts, 25
Squibb, 109
Staff Round, 12, 29, 32, 51, 87, 170
statin, 87, 90, 171, 177, 179–180, 182, 190
statin intolerance, 179, 181
statin-refractory, 181
St. Bartholomew's Hospital, 26
steatorrhoea, 30, 37
Steinberg, Dan, 53, 70, 85, 97
Steiner, Robert, 71
St. George's Hospital, 106
St. Mary's Hospital, 7, 57, 169
Stockholm, 173–174
Stoffel, Wilhelm, 118
St. Petersburg, 160, 187
St. Thomas's Hospital, 3–7, 11, 55
sucrose, 46
sudden cardiac death, 146
sugar, 48–49
sugar hypothesis, 46
Suilven, 139
Sutherland, 134

T

Taggart, Peter, 48
Takoradi, 17
tendon xanthoma, 70, 124
Test, 35, 188–189

Texas, 38–42
The Queen, Her Majesty, 119
Tobert, Jonathan, 87, 91, 180
translational research, 174
triglyceride, 52
Twain, Mark, 92, 173

U

University of Texas Southwestern Medical School, 120
Upper Falls pool, 136–138
Upper Smashie, 138–139
US Drug Enforcement Agency, 150
USSR, 159

V

Vagelos, Roy, 89
very low density lipoprotein (VLDL), 85
Vigfusson, Orri, 134
vitamin D absorption, 30, 32, 50, 190
vitamin D deficiency, 30

W

ω3 fatty acids, 81
Walton, Isaac, 189
war, 1
Wellcome Trust Centre, 113
West Africa, 21, 23
West of Scotland Coronary Primary Prevention Study (WOSCOPS), 109, 111
White, Paul Dudley, 58
WHO trial, 69, 108–109
Winneba, 19
Wood, Paul, 55–57, 65, 68
Wormwood Scrubs, 14, 28, 142
Wright, Helen Payling, 80
Wylie, George, 153

Y

Yellowstone Park, 34
Yeltsin, Boris, 159
Youmans, John, 61
Yudkin, John, 46–47, 49, 76

www.ingramcontent.com/pod-product-compliance
Lightning Source LLC
LaVergne TN
LVHW010336220926
848484LV00004BB/910